Medical Materialities

Medical Materialities investigates possible points of cross-fertilisation between medical anthropology and material culture studies, and considers the successes and limitations of both sub-disciplines as they attempt to understand places, practices, methods, and cultures of healing. The editors present and expand upon a definition of 'medical materiality', namely the social impact of the agency of often mundane, at times non-clinical, materials within contexts of health and illness, as caused by the properties and affordances of this material. The chapters address material culture in various clinical and biomedical contexts and in discussions that link the body and healing. The diverse ethnographic case studies provide valuable insight into the way cultures of medicine are understood and practised.

Aaron Parkhurst is a lecturer in Biosocial Medical Anthropology at University College London, UK, with a focus on the anthropology of the human body, and the anthropology and bioethics of emerging technology.

Timothy Carroll is a British Academy Postdoctoral Fellow in Anthropology at University College London, UK, studying end-of-life and post-mortem care amongst Orthodox Christians in Britain.

Routledge Studies in Health and Medical Anthropology

www.routledge.com/Routledge-Studies-in-Health-and-Medical-Anthropology/
book-series/RSHMA

Medical Materialities

Toward a Material Culture
of Medical Anthropology

**Edited by Aaron Parkhurst
and Timothy Carroll**

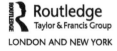

LONDON AND NEW YORK

First published 2019
by Routledge
2 Park Square, Milton Park, Abingdon, Oxon OX14 4RN

and by Routledge
52 Vanderbilt Avenue, New York, NY 10017

First issued in paperback 2020

Routledge is an imprint of the Taylor & Francis Group, an informa business

British Library Cataloguing-in-Publication Data
A catalogue record for this book is available from the British Library

Library of Congress Cataloging-in-Publication Data
A catalog record has been requested for this book

ISBN 13: 978-0-367-66288-2 (pbk)
ISBN 13: 978-1-138-31429-0 (hbk)

Typeset in Sabon
by Apex CoVantage, LLC

Contents

Figures

Contributors

Caroline Ackley received her PhD in Anthropology from University College London and is currently a Research Fellow with London School of Hygiene and Tropical Medicine. Her PhD explored Somali women's relationships with their body, other women in the community, the divine, and with their husbands. Her current research is on child and maternal health in Eastern Ethiopia. She is interested in life course development, gendered bodies and body modification, ethics and morality, post-colonialism, and the Anthropology of Islam.

Ignacia Arteaga is an affiliated lecturer and teaching associate in the Department of Social Anthropology, University of Cambridge. Her PhD (UCL) examined the material, ethical, and affective dimensions of colorectal cancer treatments, and it described the ways in which patients improvised ways of carrying on with life inside and outside a cancer clinic in London. Beyond cancer care, she is also interested in using anthropological approaches to illuminate issues of inequality, affect, and human-animal relations.

Jesse Bia is a medical anthropologist and a specialist in the Anthropology of Japan. His research expertise includes perceptions of cellular biotechnology, pluralities of Japanese medicine (including kampo), elderly healthcare, ritual pollution (kegare), bioethics, organ transplantation, and shinbutsu-shūgō. Based in the Greater Tokyo Area, his current work utilises a socio-historical methodology to examine the impacts of regenerative medicine and cellular therapies in Japanese society, focusing primarily on the experiences and narratives of patients, physicians, and nurses. He was recently hosted as a Visiting Researcher at Osaka University and conducted two years of multi-sited fieldwork sponsored by an Inoue Masaru Grant.

Timothy Carroll is a social anthropologist of material culture and conducts research amongst Eastern Orthodox Christians. Carroll's research has been conducted principally in the UK and the US, looking at Eastern Christians in Western contexts. He is currently a British Academy

Postdoctoral Fellow at University College London, studying end-of-life and post-mortem care amongst Orthodox Christians in Britain. His research engages the role of the body as a cultural artefact within medical, ritual, and art contexts. He is author of *Orthodox Christian Material Culture: Of People and Things in the Making of Heaven* (Routledge 2018).

Sophie Duckworth received her medical degree from University College London (UCL) and is currently undertaking specialist training in General Practice in the UK. Her interests are within the field of Palliative Medicine and the culture of 'care' in the clinical encounter, and she has recently completed a one-year placement in a rural community hospice in Hawke's Bay, New Zealand. She has a long-term interest in the social and palliative dimensions of tea, and she completed her MSc in Medical Anthropology at UCL in 2016. Her research examines the dimensions of 'care' expressed through the cultural practice of offering tea in hospital wards in the UK.

Sahra Gibbon is Reader in Medical Anthropology in the Department of Anthropology at University College London. She has carried out research related to genomics, health, and society in the UK, Cuba, and Brazil and has a particular interest in cancer genetics, identity, activism, and public health. Some of her major publications have focused on developments in breast cancer genetics. They include *Breast Cancer Genes and the Gendering of Knowledge: Science and Citizenship in the Cultural Context of the 'New' Genetics* (Palgrave Macmillan 2007) as well as the co-edited volume *Breast Cancer Gene Research and Medical Practices: Transnational Perspectives in the Time of BRCA* (Routledge 2014). Most recently, she has co-edited the *Routledge Handbook of Genomics, Health and Society* (2018).

Dalia Iskander is a medical anthropologist at University College London. She specialises in malaria in the Philippines and has conducted long-term fieldwork with the Pälawan indigenous community. She is particularly interested in the intersection between health practice and power as well as potential strategies to influence health practice. In her work, she has used participatory visual methodologies, namely photovoice, and evaluated how and why this methodology can potentially alter practice. She is also interested in children and young people and the role they play in ensuring their own health as well as that of their families and wider communities. She has conducted postdoctoral research on similar themes in Malaysian Borneo, where she explored the relationship between movement and malaria risk, and the UK, where she evaluated a levy on sugary drinks on consumption practices in restaurants.

David (Jeeva) Jeevendrampillai is a postdoctoral fellow at NTNU, Tronheim, Norway who specialises in the intersection between geography, architecture, and anthropology. His interests include technology, modernity, land and territoriality, the body, and anthropology of outer space. Jeevendrampillai has published his ethnographic work tracing the emergence of the local subject in liberal democracies, in particular through tracing the changing face of community organisation in London's suburbs. Following his research fellowship on planetary futures with the Institute of Advanced Studies (UCL), he is currently working on developing an anthropology of outer space through a consideration of territoriality, the body, and hegemonic narratives of the future at a planetary scale.

Roland Littlewood is a psychiatrist and anthropologist. He is Emeritus Professor of Anthropology and Psychiatry at UCL and currently Professorial Research Fellow, UCL Anthropology. He is a former President of the Royal Anthropological Institute and has conducted fieldwork in Trinidad, Haiti, Lebanon, Italy, and Albania. He has authored and edited 11 books and published over 200 papers.

Rebecca Lynch is an assistant professor (Lecturer) in Medical Anthropology at the London School of Hygiene and Tropical Medicine (LSHTM). She is interested in constructions of the body, health and illness, and risk, uncertainty, and the future, through medical, moral, and religious frameworks and interactions with the non-human (technology, protocols, bodily fluids, spirit agents, material 'stuff'). She has conducted fieldwork in Trinidad on Evangelical Christian understandings of health and the body and in the UK on biomedical and public health technologies and practices.

Aaron Parkhurst is a lecturer in Medical Anthropology at University College London (UCL) with a focus on biosocial anthropology, the anthropology of the human body, and the anthropology and bioethics of emerging technology. His work addresses men's health issues, chronic illness, and the effects of urban life on both physical and mental health, including links between depression, obesity, and blood sugar disorders. Prior to his work in London, he conducted research in Dubai with UCL and the Health Authority of Abu Dhabi (HAAD) to study indigenous understandings of health and well-being in the Arabian Gulf. His current work is focused on biosocial understandings of biomedicine and genetics, humanity's anxieties and struggles with modernity, the Anthropology of Sport, and the human body in outer space.

Kelly Fagan Robinson worked for six years in development and strategy consultancy, with several years managing NHS contracts for access to signed and spoken language interpretation. Often field-based in hospitals, she gained unique perspective into communication stresses at the care provision frontline, particularly due to clinicians' and patients' contrasting conceptions of 'bodies' and 'wellness.' She worked (2009–2014) at Deafinitely Theatre, ultimately conducting field research into deaf artists' strategies for communicating with non-deaf audiences. Her work within deaf-led welfare charities contributed to her ESRC/AHRC-funded inter-disciplinary doctoral research on interstices between public policy and deaf heritage in the UK, based at UCL Anthropology, which focused on the ways that sensorial hierarchies and communicative resources come to bear on experiences within British institutions. She is currently working with Dr Sahra Gibbon as part of the British Academy Newton Advanced Grant, examining experiences of disability and public policies in the UK and Brazil.

Graeme Were is the Chair and Professor of Anthropology in the Department of Anthropology and Archaeology at the University of Bristol. He has previously held positions at the University of Queensland, University College London, the British Museum, and Goldsmiths London. His research interests include museum anthropology, digital heritage, and material culture studies. He has a regional specialism in Papua New Guinea, where he has conducted ongoing ethnographic fieldwork since 2000, and in Vietnam, where he has collaborated with the Vietnamese Ministry of Culture, Sport and Tourism since 2013. His most recent work includes (co-edited with J.C.H. King) *Extreme Collecting: Challenging Practices for 21st Century Museums* (Berghahn, 2012).

With over a decade of experience working as a frontline healthcare prac-titioner, **Rebecca Williams** is currently undertaking an ESRC funded PhD at UCL looking at end-of-life care for terminally ill undocumented migrants in the UK. She has previously conducted research in health ser-vice community engagement, peer-led health initiatives, NHS referral process cost and patient experience, and she has undertaken extensive ethnographic research in reproductive health clinics. With a focus on the material and the body, her work critically engages with issues of access, identity, sovereignty, and care provision. Drawing from the fields of phi-losophy, anthropology, medicine, and public health, she takes seriously the idea that an interdisciplinary approach can improve health outcomes and her work actively engages with professional practice.

Acknowledgements

Medical Materialities is a project made possible by the Department of Anthropology at University College London. Specific colleagues, as well as a general atmosphere that encourages critical dialogue and opportunities for collaborative exploration of new research areas, have allowed us to develop and test the ideas that appear in this volume. Most notably, these colleagues include Susanne Küchler and Christophe Soligo as Heads of Department, Martin Holbraad as Coordinator for Reading and Research Groups, and Paul Carter-Bowman for his much-appreciated administrative help over the years.

This volume is the fruition of a two-year conversation, first organised as a Reading and Research Group (RRG), and then as a symposium. In most cases, those in regular attendance at the RRG are also contributors to the volume. Each has helped form the ideas, critiquing the general theme, and each other's specific contributions. It has been a distinct privilege and true pleasure to work with these colleagues and friends as this project developed. Similarly, we are deeply appreciative of Sahra Gibbon and Graeme Were, who graciously accepted our invitation to offer responses to the volume – adding a depth of critical insight that is a great boon.

We want to highlight, and thank, two people whose mark and influence in this volume may otherwise go unnoticed. The first is Ben Kasstan, who helped Aaron and Timothy formulate the initial concept of 'medical materialities' while in the context of editing his chapter for our previous edited volume on *Material Culture of Failure*. The second is Alison Macdonald, who has been an integral part of this conversation over the last two years, but was not able to contribute a chapter. Her contribution, though invisible, has been invaluable.

We also greatly appreciate our editors at Routledge: Louisa Vahtrick, who received Timothy's initial pitch of the idea with real enthusiasm and interest, and Katherine Ong and Marc Stratton, who have seen us through each successive stage. We also thank our anonymous reviewers for their helpful critiques and suggestions.

Timothy's involvement has been funded by the British Academy for the Humanities and Social Sciences, as part of a Postdoctoral Fellowship.

Last, and most important, we thank our families for their constant support throughout research, writing, and editing.

1 Introduction

A genealogy of medical materialities

Timothy Carroll and Aaron Parkhurst

It is important to highlight, from the outset, that Medical Anthropology and Material Culture Studies (though to a lesser degree) are projects of Social (or Sociocultural) Anthropology. The subsequent two sections frame the major movements and contributions of Medical Anthropology and Material Culture Studies as separate discourses, but the stark contrast between the two sub-disciplines – from, for example, the view of an undergraduate student – is largely an accident of module listings, not theoretical, or methodological, stance. To be sure, there are differences, and their histories of development arose from specific moments in – usually interdisciplinary – progress. It is this interdisciplinarity, and specifically the interdisciplinary partnerships characterised in each respective sub-discipline, that gives rise to the differences. Medical Anthropology, for its part, grew partly out of the work of physicians and other medical practitioners. These scholars and practitioners found partners in dialogue with social and cultural anthropologists working on ritual healing or religious cosmologies of well-being. These interdisciplinary partnerships are ongoing, and they continue to shape how Medical Anthropology exists. For its part, Material Culture Studies as it exists today is both a continuation of a long-standing aspect of Anthropology (especially in the German and American schools of practice) and a relatively new discussion, arising in response to, and negotiation around, the crisis of representation. These discourses, attending to fields of human society and cultural practice such as art, media, consumption, and the environment (both built and 'natural'), are often done in dialogue with disciplines such as Archaeology, Art History and Art Practise, Design, Media Studies, and many other, at times curious, bedfellows. When the *Journal of Material Culture* was founded, the editors specifically called it an 'undisciplined' study (Editors 1996). This undisciplined nature of Material Culture Studies has clear impact on the sort of Social Anthropology done by those in the sub-discipline, but the Material Culture being done by Anthropologists is clearly different (in method, theory, scope, etc.) from that by, for example, Historians. In each case, that is with both Medical and Material Anthropology, the kind of Social Anthropology achieved is shaped by the dialogue partners outside the discipline. As such, the project we are engaged in here is not so much about bringing two very different things together, but about asking and provoking questions, looking at what we might gain by bringing, for example, Medical Anthropology into dialogue with Art Historians, or Anthropologists of Material Culture into dialogue with Physicians.

Medical anthropology and the stuff of healing

Anthropologists have long been interested in folk medicine and healing. Indeed, the discipline has often shown how practices of healing and well-being are rarely distinct from practices of, say, witchcraft, sorcery, or spirit possession. They are interwoven in the complexity of local cosmology, and for early anthropologists, understanding 'healing' and 'medicine' was crucial in understanding the very fabric of society. Malinowski (1960 [1944]:91), for example, outlined cultural practices devoted to healing as one of his seven fundamental functions of society. Lévi-Strauss (2000 [1949]) extrapolated on functionalist anthropology by attempting to show *how* and *why* healing works through structural analysis, premised on polythetic chains of epistemology. The concept of the 'shaman' became a pivotal object of study. Many early ethnographers crucial to the development of the discipline in Britain, such as W.H.R. Rivers and Charles Seligman, were themselves practicing physicians. In this regard, the 'things' of medicine have always been present in anthropological inquiry. Objects used in healing rituals are scattered across academic departments throughout Britain and put on display in museums named after these founding academics. The Pitt Rivers museum in Oxford, for example, boasts 6,000 amulets and charms in its collection, each imbued with a unique use and social heritage.

These objects of ethnomedicine are crucial in understanding ritual healing and have been central in analysing the efficacy of symbolism, or the transitional states of rites of passage – in this case, between sickness and health, or life and death. Medical materials are often key within ethnography, but the way they are analysed is often quite limited. Healing objects are often imbued with symbolic meaning in analysis of medical rituals. Victor (1964) and Edith (1994) Turner, for example, have written extensively on Ihamba rituals among the Ndembu in order to theorise how communities are made and healed within the liminal phases of ritual. The Ihamba is understood as both the tooth of the hunter and the spirit of that hunter. It is a symbol of masculinity, but it is also regarded as a literal ancestor. When illness occurs, the Ihamba can be appeased. After a successful ritual, the tooth becomes a sacred talisman, guiding its wearer in hunting. Similarly, amulets and charms devoted to warding off the evil eye are plentiful across the Mediterranean and Islamic world. Analysis of their efficacy focuses on the representation of gaze, or counter gaze, to the conscious or subconscious emotions present in public interaction – the jealous or malevolent 'stare' that causes illness and malaise. The amulets take on many forms: a striking blue glass eye with dilated pupils, a form of a hand with the eye placed in the palm, or perhaps a Christian cross with the eye at its centre. Each refers back to the eye with perhaps different socio-religious aesthetics. Herzfeld (1981) has pointed out that, despite being a well-established folk category of disease, the history of the evil eye in Anthropology has been limited to the eye as a symbolic category in and of itself. He argues, ultimately, that the evil eye must be understood in terms of larger semiotic and symbolic systems. This call echoes the Turners' call for situating symbolic efficacy in wider relational and communal (and perhaps moral) systems, themes that are so crucial and prominent in Medical Anthropology. However, it fails to address the material affordances of the objects it analyses – the amulets that heal, the air through which the malignant gaze takes flight and, of course, the biological eye itself, of the individual who stares, and of the individual who can see the public eyes upon them.

Mary Douglas (2003 [1966]) has helped forward this call for wider symbolic systems by asking *where* illness is located within socio-cultural epistemology. She frames her argument in comparison to the 'medical materialism,' proposed by the philosopher William James, which rationalises religious phenomena (a vision, for instance, or food prohibitions) as the result of medical phenomena (an aneurysm or psychedelic episode, for example, or hygiene needs). 'There is no objection to this approach,' argues Douglas,

> unless it excludes other interpretations. Most primitive peoples are medical materialists in an extended sense, in so far as they tend to justify their ritual actions in terms of aches and pains which would afflict them should the rites be neglected.

However, she does dismiss the position, saying, 'By the time I have finished with ritual danger I think no one should be tempted to take such beliefs at face value' (2003 [1966]: 33). The opposing view, that 'primitive ritual' has no relation to concepts of health, she equally dismisses. Ultimately, for Douglas, *where* illness lies is 'out of place.' Douglas asks her readers to consider the context in which objects are placed as the fundamental feature of what constitutes dirt and pollution. In Douglas' hierarchical view of culture, objects are best understood as being entirely subject to the context in which they are embedded. Their categorisations as clean or dirty are dependent on how they speak towards the systems of relations in which they are embedded, and because all dirt is relational, no object can be intrinsically dirty. This emphasis on symbolic systems has helped shape the way that materials are understood in Medical Anthropology, and in many regards have helped highlight the complexity of healing objects and practices. Under Douglas' thinking, the same objects that are culturally taboo, impure, or dangerous, might also be used for healing – their danger gives them power. However, the emphasis on the context of materials has in some regards left the objects out of analysis. Somewhere between William James and Mary Douglas, a more holistic appraisal of taboo and social phenomena is needed – an approach that integrates the material constitution of the object, and links that within the sociality of the taboo. For Douglas, the dirtiness of objects becomes almost accidental.

In the 1970s, Medical Anthropology began to take its hold as a sub-discipline within Anthropology. While ethnomedicine had long been a focus within Euro-American Anthropology, thinkers such as Arthur Kleinman, Byron Good, Leon Eisenberg, and Roland Littlewood led a call for Anthropology to turn its gaze on the cultures of Euro-American Medical systems, recognising biomedicine as its own powerful cultural system (Littlewood 1992; Kleinman et al. 1978; Kleinman 1980; Good 1993). This important work focused on the ways in which biomedicine is informed by the biases, assumptions, and power structures woven throughout any society in which biomedicine is practised. The analysis of patient-clinician interactions gave rise to calls for and critiques of cultural competency in the clinic (Kleinman and Benson 2006; Singer 1995; Lewis-Fernández et al. 2014). Similar to the ways a relativistic stance has helped shape other social domains, the concept and implementation of cultural competence in the clinic is multifaceted. Hospital ethnography asks for physicians to pay heed to their patients' understanding of illness and health and the body (cultural or other) to provide better health provision and have more impact upon health outcomes, while other critiques of biomedicine show the inherent biases, assumptions, racism, and patriarchal influence embedded within the practice of medical diagnosis and pharmacological prescription (Lipsedge and Littlewood 2005; Fadiman 1997).

In recent years, cultural competency within hospital ethnography has begun to re-examine healing as situated not only in doctor provision and patient reception, but in the practice and enactment of the body in medicine (Mol 2002, 2008, for example), and more concretely, as situated in the practice of quotidian life (Mattingly 1994; Tropea 2012; Calabrese 2013). These models of 'therapeutic emplotment' afford discussions on material culture that are more absent in traditional hospital ethnography. Anthropologists might traditionally have examined post-surgery – physical therapy, for example – through the power structures embedded in the clinical encounter, or the culture clashes between incommensurable or conflicting definitions of disability or illness. However, models of therapeutic emplotment afford anthropological discussion on the 'making of a person's reality' (Calabrese 2013:42) through their interaction with the objects and techniques that get them through their day – a comb, for example, as an instrument that requires bodily technique, but affords one an opportunity to present oneself to a family member or friend (Mattingly 1994). Similarly, Material Culture Studies has also recently turned to these quotidian interactions of subtle health making, showing how material interactions are woven into various situated performances of care, such as the use of hand sanitisers, soaps, and gloves (Pink et al. 2014).

Drugs and other pharmaceutical materials have justifiably been an important focus in Medical Anthropology because of the various politics, power structures, and practices that ethnographic focus on pharma brings to light. Anthropologists have been fascinated by the dual nature of the 'pharmakon' as both remedy and poison and have shown how this ambiguity affords meaning-making in different contexts (e.g. Martin 2006, 2007; Whyte et al. 2002). Borrowing from material culture analytics proposed by Appadurai (1986), Whyte et al. have compiled ethnographies that outline the social and biographical lives of medicines (2002), demonstrating the role of *Materia Medica* as solving social problems, the role of prescription as a social and political act, and distribution and consumption as medicalised and cultural processes. The ambiguous nature of the pharmakon also affords important debate in bioethics, transnational processes, and structural inequality, what Petryna and Kleinman refer to as 'the pharmaceutical nexus' (2006).

This understanding of the pharmakon relies on the material good to be the focal point through which social processes intersect. For example, they highlight how important drugs that are developed and manufactured in the US are a small fraction of the cost in Canada, which provides subsidised healthcare for its citizens through social security. Inequity within American health insurance structures force citizens in the US to cross the border to purchase life-saving drugs, often from unregulated markets. American pharmaceutical companies concerned over loss of profit then threaten Canadian policy makers by withholding distribution of new drugs unless the Canadian government regulates the sale of drugs in Canada to US citizens. Here, Petryna and Kleinman show how the pharmaceutical nexus highlights how

> the astonishing social logic that results in drugs produced by American pharmaceutical firms costing less outside the United States is hardly challenged by economists and policy analysts since it is rational in the global system of trade, but it needs to be understood anthropologically as a telling critique of what has become cultural common-sense about global trade.
>
> (2006:15)

More recently, Hardon and Moyer continue these important discussions through diverse ethnographies that further complicate the nexus, showing how anthropological analysis highlights 'the need to incorporate in our analytical frameworks the creative agency of the users of medical technologies, the particularities of local markets and care constellations, class hierarchies, social relations and family dynamics' (2014:112). Other ethnographies focus on drugs and other medical materials as context to understand the biases and politics within bioethics and international regulation. Bharadwaj's (2013) research on stem cell clinics in India, for example, uses stem cell research to tease out subaltern practice, complicating international regulation and asking questions on who benefits and who is disadvantaged.

The ethnographies delicately elucidate important social structures, and they provide an evidence base for addressing imbalance within healthcare provision and gaps within cultures of care. However, these pieces of research understand medical materials as objects and ideas upon which social relations are mapped. Emily Martin (2006, 2007) takes this further in her work on pharmaceutical persons. She writes that drugs are,

> inanimate objects that cannot literally speak, think or feel, pharmaceutical marketers and advertisers attempt to invest (them) with attributes to make it possible to think of them as 'persons,' as if they were social beings with individual personalities.
>
> (2007:150)

Indeed, pharmaceutical and advertising companies may very well take that approach, and it has important implications for cultures of medicalisation. The ways in which people attribute meaning to drugs, or place politics and personalities to pills and technologies, is diverse and fascinating. However, what these approaches fail to address is the materiality of the objects themselves, those properties of the pharmakon that afford and inform social relations. Rather than understand pills, for example, as only 'invested' with attributes by users, this volume interrogates the material constitution of medical objects and substances, exploring how the properties and affordances of the material impact upon the social and medical contexts. In doing so, these chapters – to varying degrees – unpack how the eventual processes of investiture may emerge and how symbolic or broader epistemological aspects of the pharmaceutical nexus are – like Gell's (1998) art nexus – grounded in and around the object.

In thinking about the nexus and the growth of invested meanings in and around the object, it is important to highlight the layers of complexity in, to continue the example, the pharmakon. While the 'active chemical agent' of a pill is, ostensibly, the thing that 'does' something, it can be problematic to ascribe agency to the chemical. (For more on the terminology here, see below.) As we know from work on placebo (e.g. Moerman 2002), and nocebo (e.g. Požgain et al. 2014; Justman 2016), there need not be an active, medicinal chemical to produce health benefits or speed a patient's decline. However, as Moerman shows, the 'meaning response' is linked to the accidental qualities of the pharmacological entity. In a classical Geertzian sense, the meaning is derived from the 'web of symbols' (Geertz 2004 [1966]) constitutive of culture. But the question remains: why? Why these accidental qualities, why these effects or, phrased a different way, why this material and why this materiality?

Material culture studies and 'materiality'

The discipline of Anthropology grew alongside the colonial expansion and development of national collections. Museums such as the Pitt Rivers, the British Museum and the Horniman in Britain or the Peabody and Field

Museums in the US, and various museums of ethnography, ethnology, or humanity across Europe (the names of which often changed) held collections of artefacts brought back from distant lands or, in the North American context, from indigenous peoples. In this context, early social theorists studied the art objects of the cultural 'other' as part of the budding discipline of Anthropology. The extent to which material culture was part of the genesis of Anthropology can be seen, for example, in Lewis Henry Morgan's (1877) *Ancient Society*, where the techniques of production and various modes of technological advancement of various peoples were used as evidence within evolutionary models of human development.

The place of techniques of cultural production also became central within the anthropological investigation of art practice. In North America, cultural anthropologists like Franz Boas were actively engaged in the formal analysis of both people (1891, 1898, 1915) and things (1897, 1916, 1927). The formal analysis of people, specifically the phrenological measurement and categorisation of indigenous peoples, is part of anthropology's history that today we would rather forget. However, the darker side of the science of phrenology, and its use in the hegemonic and racist evaluation of 'primitive' peoples, is important to remember. The assumption that the 'inside' of the person could be known via outside visible markers linked the biological body with the essence of the person. At the time, the prominent view concerning the unilinear progression of human cognition also meant that such 'primitive' peoples, as well as those in Europe with less desirable facial features, were assumed less intelligent. The link between mind and body, as a visible correspondence, also appears in the analysis of 'primitive' art as conducted by Boas (1955 [1927]). His formal analysis of art, conducted at a huge comparative scale of the Pacific Rim, was carried out alongside phrenological analysis. And, too, the link between cognition and physically visible elements is explicit. However, for Boas, who argued against racialisation and the claims to racial superiority (1915), both indicate that the 'savage' mind and the 'civilised' (to use Morgan's lowest and highest categories) alike had the same cognitive capacity.

In the American school, objects continued to hold an important place within cultural Anthropology. Alfred Irving Hallowell argued that

> object orientation likewise provides the ground for an intelligible interpretation of events in the behavioural environment on the basis of traditional assumptions regarding the nature and attributes of the objects involved and implicit or explicit dogmas regarding the 'cause' of events.
> (2002:19)

This is a rich methodological position and clearly signals the possibilities of what has become known as a material culture approach. The possibility of sociocultural analysis via object orientation is evident in vast literature, and a variety of interpretational models have arisen. Most common within sociocultural anthropology are approaches such as symbolic or semiotic anthropology, which, each in their own way, attempt to place objects (and language, and social practice, etc.) within frameworks of representational indication, such that the object stands in for or points towards part of the system of beliefs and symbols so central to a Geertzian definition of culture (cf. Geertz 1966).

This movement towards symbolic or semiotic representation, however, lost sight of a key aspect of Boas' perspective. The link between the visible and the internal, between the artefactual surface and the cognitive content, was not, for Boas, only representational. The artistic virtuosity – that is the technically advanced skill and the even regularity of design execution – was not principally a question of *what* the California First Nations Peoples thought about, but *how* they thought. It is also important to note that this 'how' of thinking was not that of a diagram, but a discourse thinking *with* materials. Boas' example (1955:20) of a weaver feeling, sensing, knowing the reeds with which she works speaks of the impact, or at least the potential impact, of materials on cultural production.

The methodological holism of anthropology and the anthropocentrism of social theory has become a continuous discourse within the field. The degree to which human will and intention, as knowing subject, drive human culture, versus the impact of objects, inanimate or otherwise, within society is an important place of ongoing theoretical concern. Early models of systems, incorporating human and non-human entities, such as Bateson's cybernetic approach, emphasised the feedback loops whereby social action and human behaviour is informed and shaped by ecological behaviour (Bateson 1972, 1987). The degree to which people make things and things make people became an important guiding trope for material culture studies, and the possibility of studying things as means to understand people and as part of human society and culture also offered a useful means to obviate the political tensions rising to the fore in the second half of the twentieth century.

With the slow implementation of decolonisation and the growth of the civil rights movement, the legitimacy of the established Euro-American academy and their universalist claim to knowledge was called into question. The crisis of representation challenged, and rightly so, the White male gaze and its authority to speak about and interpret the cultural 'other.' While active social scientific analysis of indigenous peoples became politically suspect, and especially in the US the study of First Nations Peoples became legally constrained, a new interest in material culture, as a specific methodological approach within (and sometimes separate from) broader sociocultural anthropology was born. Archaeology (which in the US is usually a subdiscipline of Anthropology) helped shift the focus of anthropological investigation from the living cultural practices to the objects. It was, as Fowles (2016) argues, politically safer to speak about things than people.

The other important factor in the development of material culture, as it is known today, is seen in the interdisciplinary work by those like Daryll

Forde and Peter Ucko. Forde, himself trained in both British Social Anthropology and American Cultural Anthropology, made a point of establishing the department of anthropology at UCL with a mind to the broad-based holism of anthropology. With the appointment of archaeologist Peter Ucko, Forde institutionalised teaching of material culture in anthropology, 'the term material culture was adopted to emphasize an approach which combined the study of both contemporary and past non-literate cultures from the point of view of the material record' (Rowlands 1983:15). In Ucko's own estimation, the 'one thing which distinguishes the study of material culture from most other aspects of anthropological investigation [. . .] is that its data are manufactured objects, the result of some technological process' (1969:29). The benefit, in this view, of material culture within anthropology was that objects endured through time, allowing a synchronic analysis of cultural phenomenon. Objects could be revisited and used to revisit old questions with new analytical and scientific advancements. The formal, and morphological, analysis of collections and archaeological finds afforded the groundwork to address large guiding themes about human variation and culture change.

By the 1980s, however, as it became more difficult to speak about the (post-)colonial other, the increased application of anthropological methods 'at home' saw the application of material culture methods to contemporary communities, literate or not. Influenced by French sociology and philosophy, anthropology's historic focus on the distant other began to fade. By the end of the twentieth century, works by Appadurai (1986), Gell (1998), Latour (1991, 1993, 1999), Miller (1997), and many others – as well as the founding of the *Journal of Material Culture* in 1996 – placed objects (or things, or any number of other similar terms, see below) at the centre of the analytical focus. Because of the common ground, or rather overlapping areas of interest, between anthropology, archaeology, and art history, intellectual traditions in the latter, as well as in art criticism and aesthetics, became influential in the material culture approach to art and the agency of things.

In the spirit of Forde's holism, the founding editors of the *Journal of Material Culture* specifically identified material culture studies as 'undisciplined.' They defend this, saying, 'We argue then that being undisciplined can be highly productive if it leads us to focus upon areas that established disciplines have ignored because of boundary constraints' (Editors 1996:13). Material culture studies has, at least in Britain, always been something of an intellectual safe haven for experimentalism and the disciplinarily disaffected (Rowlands 1983; Editors 1996; Buchli 2002). While the intellectual heritage from archaeology and morphological analysis is still palpable within much present-day works of material culture, the emphasis on non-literate and historic peoples has, at least within anthropology, largely given way to the ethnographic study of contemporary populations. The emphasis on art (broadly conceived) and technology is, however, still quite dominant, and the border grounds between anthropology and STS studies, art history, design, human geography, and other social scientific disciplines is often difficult to distinguish. In many cases, key thinkers – such as Michel Foucault or Bruno Latour – are read by scholars across the spectrum, but read differently, or focusing on different works, by scholars in different fields.

As it relates to our present focus, the critical contribution from material culture studies arises in the shift of focus from studying object as means to understand cultural difference to the study of object as participant within the ongoing production of human society. Works like *Art and Agency* (Gell 1998) and *Aramis* (Latour 1993), amongst others, provoked important questions concerning the place of objects (or more properly technological systems, in Latour's case) within human society. Gell's final monograph outlines how human agency may come to be concretised within art-like artefacts, thereby rendering them 'secondary agents.' The possibility of objects having agency of their own to act in the world, separate from their artist-crafter, opens up important possibilities. This position has been critiqued both for removing human agency from the centre focus (Morphy 2009) and for granting humans too much of a central role (Ingold 2010b). At the heart of this disagreement is the role of intention within action, and the degree to which humans and non-humans may have or lack intention.

Agency, roughly defined as the capacity to intentionally effect change, belongs to entities (human or otherwise) who act in the world knowingly and intentionally. Alongside the term 'agent' – indicating the person or object that acts with intention – other terms such as 'actor' or 'actant' may also be used. This later distinction, between actor and actant comes originally from the folklorist Vladimir Propp (1968), who is most famous for his analysis of Russian folk narratives. Actor and actant, in this context, are principally functional categories. An actant performs certain functions within the narrative plot. Put in today's terminology of video and role-playing games, an actant is an NPC (non-playing character). An actor, by contrast, is a more developed character, having personality and a key contributing part to play within the plot development. The actor/actant language tends to focus on the function within a system – for example, of a character in a folktale, or a microscope in the production of scientific knowledge. For Latour, the functional role of the actant becomes that of mediation or translation: effectively the movement of something from one status to another. Agentive language differs from this approach by focusing on the role of intentional action or, particularly in Gell's case, the social impact of the interpretation of intention.

This aspect of interpretation becomes very important in exploring what art and other forms of social action do. In terms of causal sequencing, it matters less what Person A intends to do to Person B than what Person B interprets Person A to have intended. In the immediacy of social interaction, Person B will respond to Person A based on their intuitive, immediate interpretation of Person A's action. It may or may not be correct, but it is this attribution of agency that guides the reaction. What is clear from across the ethnographic witness is that humans, in many varieties of ways, attribute agentive action to non-human entities. In many cases, these entities are objects, either organic or mineral substances or crafted artefacts. What becomes interesting in these cases is how such objects and artefacts are seen to be agentive. What about the materials in question – be it their design, or the ingredients used – allows them to become actants and actors within human society?

The other language often used to address the relation between objects (or environments) and human action or experience is that of affordances. Affordances, as coined by Gibson (1979), describes what the object (and specifically the surface of the object) enables the person to do with or against it. A chair affords someone to sit upon it. The properties of a material will afford different kind of action, and while a wood chair and one made of polystyrene may appear the same, the second may collapse under weight. What is particularly interesting for our purposes here is that the language of affordances – building upon both the material properties of the object and the social, historical, and narrative associations bound up into the object – can be used either to avoid the language of agency or to be paired with it. The division, in this regard, lies in an ambiguity in Gibson's own writing as to if affordances are (at least predominantly) socially ascribed or somehow inherent in the objects.

This question of material inherency – that is, to what degree is the social capital of objects the result of their physical essence as opposed to the web of symbols and interpretations – is a large problem that comes to the fore in interdisciplinary discussions around materials, such as is seen in this volume. The contributing authors, to varying degrees, point to a variety of positions along a continuum. For all the claims to cultural relativity held by Anthropology, it is hard to deny that a disease entity has a physical effect on the human body, and thereby becomes (at least) an actant within human society. Medical implants, microorganisms, chemical or ritual substances, and any number of other things entering into, or into contact with, the human body; and each offer surfaces with their own affordances – some known some unanticipated and misunderstood. As Sontag has argued at length (1978, 1989), the metaphors by which we understand disease has a lasting impact on the social life of the sick and the health protocols by which we help (or hinder) them.

Another set of terminology that has, in material culture studies, an important role in how the relations between people and the stuff of our environment is understood is that of object, thing, artefact, material, and stuff. There is some variation across the literature as to how these terms are understood, and within this volume we have left it to the author to define how these terms are used, if at all. However, it can be helpful to highlight some of the implications of these terms. 'Object,' which we have used earlier somewhat indiscriminately, usually carries the connotation of being in relation to a subject. Something is an object if it is in relation to a subject, even if that subject may not be explicitly spoken of in the context. The other common usage, following from Peircean semiotics, is that the object is the actual substance (event or artefact) of signification. That is to say, a Peircean object is the empirically observable aspect of sign-making and sign-interpretation. This aspect of Peircean semiotics has, as Milton Singer (1980; cf. Mertz 2007) notes, allowed for a more empirically grounded enquiry into how meaning is made and circulated than has, by contrast, Saussurean semiology. The second term is 'thing.' Thing, for its part, usually carries the implication of process. The Heideggerian argument, linking thing to the Old German *dine*, highlights that thing has the 'meaning of a gathering specifically for the purpose of dealing with a case or matter' (Heidegger 1971:173). The explicit telos of thing, in this case, is often rejected – by, for example, Ingold (2010b) – but the processual nature of the gerund is maintained. Whereas the object is in a specific position in relation to the subject, the thing may be open ended, changing, multiple. Added to this list is 'artefact,' and the quality thereof: artefactual. An artefact is something made, in its usage there is often the implication of time and duration. It is worth highlighting that these are not mutually exclusive terms, and a thing may move from one object position to another, and that change may be in relation to its artefactual nature – it breaking or being redesigned – or due to it being gifted to another person (i.e. a different subject).

The framing of how we understand and speak about stuff – used as a generic and broad category – as an object, a thing, or an artefact casts that within specific kinds of social relations. Material is, ultimately, a social category – with terms like 'physical' as a point further down the line, outside, or before, sociality. One of the questions provoked within this volume is how the materials of medicine may be understood when investigated with explicit attention to the kind, duration, and texture of its relation to the human subjects within the medical context.

This crucial aspect of relationality – which anchors this interdisciplinary project in Social Anthropology – also offers an insight into the issue at hand while seeking to answer the question of material inherency. To take a comparison from art, Wassily Kandinsky (2008 [1911]), in discussing the role of colour and form and its capacity to evoke response within a person, offers a model that resonates surprisingly well with Gibson's affordance. He argues for the 'psychic effect' of colour, saying, 'The soul being one with the body, the former may well experience a psychic shock, caused by association acting on the latter' (2008:59). He suggests, similarly to Douglas' idea of 'natural symbol' (1970), that this effect arises from the association between, for example, red and fire, but also admits that the effect of a given colour is not universally observed across the animals and plants (Kandinsky 2008:61). He maintains, however, that 'no more sufficient, in the psychic sphere, is the theory of association. Generally speaking, colour is a power which directly influences the soul.' And using an analogy from music, he continues, 'Colour is the keyboard, the eyes are the hammers, the soul is the piano with many strings. The artist is the hand which plays, touching one key or another, to cause vibrations in the soul' (2008:61–62). Both Gibson's and Kandinsky's models situate the effectual impact of the object (be it chairs or paintings) in the capacity of the surface to do something to the soul/person directly. While both admit the influence of social, historical narrative interpretations, each supersede these extrapolations with the properties of the material object. Kandinsky, however, concludes that 'it is evident therefore that colour harmony must rest only on a corresponding vibration in the human soul' (2008:62); subsequently, he concludes the same in regards to form (2008:67) and object (2008:71). The effect of the thing rests not in the thing alone, nor in the socially attributed meanings; rather, effect rests in the harmony between the person and the thing.

A definition of medical materiality

In this vein, medical materialities is a framework for investigating the harmonic resonances and proportions held between and within the materials of medicine and the materials of the human body. It is also a framework for analysing and reframing the quotidian materials of society – bread, streets, buildings, cloth, for example – as having medical sociality. Material is inherently social, and materiality is the effects – specifically the social impact – of that material. As Tilley (2007) has summarised, material : materiality :: social : sociality (cf. Carroll et al. 2017:5). The theoretical presupposition held within the concept of medical materiality is, then, that the physical, the biological, the medical, the material, the social, the symbolic are held together within the context of care provision, well-being, and health intervention. In this way, a medical materiality is inherently biosocial. To isolate one of these aspects without the others will lose sight of the ways in which 'relations between relations' (Gell 1998:215), that is the harmony between parts, and across genre (between bodies, or between the human and non-human), are the means to accomplishing health and well-being.

The chapters in this volume each engage this concept – or, more appropriately, a field of possibility – in their own way. The unique angles, emphases, and interpretations do, however, have some common themes. The most obvious is the body, as a material object – either in its unitary operation or in the textures and variation in its internal composition. Closely coupled to this is the somatic capacity of the body to sense the world, and the world to touch the body. This capacity of material to touch, and the specific nature of that touch, also brings to the fore the theme of agency and action. Whether ascribed intention or framed in terms of chemical potency or the affordances of matter, the capacity of the material to act upon the world – be it by design, or in excessive and unanticipated ways – is at the heart of this volume. The issue of technology is also a common theme, but one that comes to the fore less in this collection than one might expect given the extensive exploration in STS studies and (especially francophone) anthropology. This is, in large part, because the nature of medical materialities as a biosocial investigation of the material culture of medical and health contexts invites an appraisal of the material ecology at a level closer to the constituent elements of the matter, before – and, in some cases, problematising – the larger epistemological and sociocultural nature of the technologies of which this material is part. This is a biosocial approach that emphasises the fact that the bio is itself a material, and material is inherently social.

The chapters are roughly organised in three parts, though there are themes – both those highlighted earlier and others – that cross cut the collection and would allow for alternative orders. Part I, on Flesh and Fluids, includes chapters that consider the fleshiness of the body itself and its substances as this, often messy, aspect of human health comes entangled in medical contexts. This begins with Chapter 2, by Rebecca Lynch, discussing the relationship between the flesh of the body and the surgical mesh used to help repair vaginal walls and urinary tracts. Lynch investigates the point where flesh and mesh meet, and the ways these materials integrate into mesh-flesh – a process full of variables including natural, social, cultural, political, and economic influences. In Chapter 3, Ignacia Arteaga examines the control of faecal matter, and the issues around stoma bags, in order to offer a critique of the notion of 'adjustment' – widely used by clinical practitioners. Arteaga's argument also highlights the partial nature of Douglas' (and wider symbolic anthropology's) understanding of the unclean 'dirt,' and brings into focus the material and infrastructural ways that the polluted individual comes to understand their own dirtiness. She argues, ultimately, that cancer sufferers can better negotiate the psychological challenges of life with stomas when the material concerns of the stoma are addressed. Caroline Ackley, in Chapter 4, considers both the flow of liquid and trapped liquid in the context of female genital cutting (FGC) practices in Somaliland. Ackley argues that FGC cannot be seen as an isolated incidence but must rather be taken as something which changes and develops with the life stages of the girls and women involved; she argues that the physical folding in and opening up of the labia mirrors the complex sociality of women in Somaliland. In Chapter 5, Rebecca Williams investigates the role of sperm in the medical practices of infertility diagnosis and the gender performances of the men coming to recognise their own infertility. Williams argues that, contrary to the anticipated new forms of social identity made possible through IVF and other reproductive technologies, at least in the andrology clinic, new technological interventions are routinely marshalled in order to maintain very normative heterosexual notions of masculinity and fatherhood.

Part II, on the Infrastructures of Care, includes chapters that examine the infrastructures, both official and supplementary, that exist within medical care provision and its governmentality. In Chapter 6, Aaron Parkhurst follows the health screening that each migrant to Dubai must undergo and considers the issues of control and unknowing that exist in a context where a failed test results in deportation. Parkhurst argues that 'following the object' is not always sufficient and instead focuses on the material disjunctures experienced by migrant labourers as their passports, blood samples, and x-ray results are separated from them. Sophie Duckworth, in Chapter 7, unpacks tea-making practices in a British Hospice setting, where the warmth of the tea operates as a materially sensuous, but partible, object that lets the warmth of compassionate care be given to the patients and the bereaved. Duckworth argues that tea becomes the material expression of time and compassionate care, allowing for presence and comfort to be felt within the hospice ward. Jesse Bia, then, in Chapter 8, looks at a recent shift in Japanese conceptions of soybeans within the context of an ageing population and social conceptions of regenerative medicine. Bia argues that the understandings of soybeans and *in vivo* regenerative medicine, and the need for a super-aged population to be sustained in good health, has shifted traditional rites from bringing luck to bringing health. In Chapter 9, the last of Part II, Kelly Fagan Robinson unpacks the process of applying for disability support in the UK and shows how the material of the government paperwork is not compatible with the spacetime of a profoundly deaf applicant. Fagan Robinson argues that the failure of the claims-form to allow for the mode of communication and knowledge production used by the deaf applicant means that the government's method of supporting those with specific needs is ultimately undone by insurmountable gaps in communication.

Part III, on Health Publics, examines the ways of understanding health and health provision within larger publics and the ways these link with larger cosmologies and epistemological frameworks. Roland Littlewood, in Chapter 10, outlines the relationship towards 'nature' expressed by a new religious movement in Trinidad, examining how the dirt, the garden vegetables, and the group's perception of the town folk can be seen to situate health in relation to the earth. Littlewood argues that his Trinidadian interlocutors address the materiality of 'Earth' as a 'floating signifier,' ultimately showing how nature is reframed as an arch-typical 'life.' Disease and misfortune are, then, caused by material forms that 'tap' the energy of nature, creating 'anti-life.' He shows how this balance is both informed by, and reproduces, a purposeful inversion of normative Trinidadian values. David Jeevendrampillai, in Chapter 11, then explores the relationship between a suburban community group in South London and a local water filtration bed, highlighting the somatisation of local landscape and the anxiety about the future, such that the health of the local body is bound up within urban planning and development. Jeevenrampillai argues that cases of ill health, such as shown here, are not simply incidental to the process of being a good modern subject. They are also symptomatic of the demand made upon the citizen who is made responsible for the urban space in which he or she lives, and yet relatively powerless to effect it. In Chapter 12, Timothy Carroll traces the historical development of frankincense from antiquity through to its contemporary usage in Orthodox Christianity in order to show how material substances play a role in how medical notions of health of the body are in close dialogue with religious notions of health and well-being. Carroll argues that the specific affordances of the person, the body, and the medical material reveal important insight into how and why certain substances are able to facilitate health. In doing so, he shows how notions of healing can be better understood by a careful examination of how materials move in and through the human body. In the final ethnographic contribution, Chapter 13, Dalia Iskander discusses the impact of a photovoice project on Malaria in the Philippines and shows how children use the photographic technology to help effect change within the rural population. Iskander argues for a reappraisal of how culture change around health issues is affected by the material aspects of education programs, highlighting that it is not 'voice,' but rather the materiality of the photos, their performance, and the ability to capture and manipulate images that affords changing perceptions of disease prevention.

The ethnographic contributions are then followed by two Responses. The first is by Sahra Gibbon who, writing as a medical anthropologist whose work is principally situated in genomics and post-genomics in Brazil and the UK, unpacks some of the implications of 'medical materialities' being framed as a 'biosocial' concept (see earlier). In doing so, she also voices an important cautionary insight, highlighting how such a framework – situated as it is across and between the biological sciences and sociocultural interpretations – can fall prey to over-interpretation and the political negotiations of promissory hope. Gibbon then thinks through the BRCA (Breast Cancer) gene, from her own research, through the perspective of medical materialities and discusses the instability of the material as an 'object' in tension between the medical scientific community and the wider social and medical contexts. The final contribution to the volume is by Graeme Were, whose research in Melanesia and Vietnam has focused largely on museum collections, the politics and history of such collections, and the social contexts from which they were sourced. In Were's response, he argues for the importance of the anthropological focus on the 'thing,' and highlights the rich methodological and analytical potential in the concept of 'medical materialities.' Looking at the history of collections, Were suggests that Henry Wellcome stands as a forbearer to the work of this volume – a salient observation, and it is no coincidence, considering this volume has been developed in the shadow of the Wellcome Collection here in London. Were ends his response working through some of the implications of what a medical materialities approach would look like in some of his earlier work, specifically in relation to the kapkap of New Ireland.

The two Responses also bring to the foreground another theme of this volume, which runs through each of the chapters. This theme revolves around the question of the 'object' and its stability. And while this may not sound immediately like a theme of medical concern, at heart it is. As Gibbon argues, the social scientific tendency to reify the object as a stable entity does have implications on how the body, the gene, and other medical artefacts are understood. While there have been critical movements away from the concept of the 'object' altogether (Ingold 2007, 2010a,b), or to recognise its instability and flux (e.g. Tilley 2007; Were 2013), or to highlight the huge social labour and infrastructure required to maintain an 'object' in its position (Domínguez Rubio 2016) – the implications for medical materials still demands investigation. Indeed, the future of biosocial inquiry, in both social science and biomedicine, may very well require such questions be asked (Ingold and Palsson 2013). What the nature of the medical material is, and how the boundedness, duration, or classification of any particular object (or substance) of investigation rests, is an integral question throughout each chapter. As a result, each contribution also offers novel ways to conceive of and analyse the objects of medicine, health, and well-being and their medical materialities.

References

Appadurai, Arjun (1986). *The Social Life of Things: Commodities in Cultural Perspective*. Cambridge: Cambridge University Press.

Bateson, Gregory (1972). *Steps to an Ecology of Mind: Collected Essays in Anthropology, Psychiatry, Evolution, and Epistemology*. Chicago: University of Chicago Press.

Bateson, Gregory (1987). The Model. In G. Bateson and M.C. Bateson (Eds.), *Angels Fear: Toward an Epistemology of the Sacred*. London: Bantam Books, 36–49.

Bharadwaj, Aditya (2013). Subaltern biology? Local biologies, Indian Odysseys, and the pursuit of human embryonic stem cell therapies. *Medical Anthropology* 32(4):359–373, DOI: 10.1080/01459740.2013.787533.

Boas, Franz (1891). Physical characteristics of the Indians of the North Pacific coast. *The American Anthropologist* 4:25–32.

Boas, Franz (1897). The decorative art of the Indians of the North Pacific coast. *Bulletin of the AMNH 9*, article 10:123–176.

Boas, Franz (1898). The growth of Toronto children. Chapter XXXIV. *Education Report 1896–97*. Washington D.C.

Boas, Franz (1915). *Race and Nationality*. New York: American Association for International Conciliation.

Boas, Franz (1916). Representative Art of Primitive People. In Frederick Webb Hodge (Ed.), *Holmes Anniversary Volume; Anthropological Essays Presented to William Henry Holmes in Honor of His Seventieth Birthday*, December 1, 1916. Washington, DC: J.W. Bryan Press, 18–23.

Boas, Franz (1955 [1927]). *Primitive Art*. Toronto: Dover Publications, Inc.

Buchli, Victor (2002). Introduction. In V. Buchli (Ed.), *The Material Culture Reader*. Oxford: Berg, 1–22.

Calabrese, Joseph (2013). *A Different Medicine: Postcolonial Healing in the Native American Church*. Oxford: Oxford University Press.

Carroll, Timothy, David Jeevandrampillai and Aaron Parkhurst (2017). Introduction: Toward a General Theory of Failure. In T. Carroll, D. Jeevandrampillai, A. Parkhurst and J. Shackelford (Eds.), *Material Culture of Failure: When Things Do Wrong*. London: Bloomsbury.

Domínguez Rubio, Fernando (2016). On the discrepancy between objects and things: An ecological approach. *Journal of Material Culture* 21(1):59–86.

Douglas, Mary (1970). *Natural Symbols*. London: Cresset Press.

Douglas, Mary (2003 [1966]). *Purity and Danger: An Analysis of Concepts of Pollution and Taboo*. London: Routledge.

Editors (1996). Editorial. *Journal of Material Culture* 1(1):5–14.

Fadiman, A. (1997). *The Spirit Catches You and You Fall Down: A Hmong Child, Her American Doctors, and the Collision of Two Cultures*. London: Macmillan.

Fowles, Severin (2016). The perfect subject (postcolonial object studies). *Journal of Material Culture* 21(1):9–27.

Geertz, Clifford (2004 [1966]). Religion as a Cultural System. In M Banton (Ed.), *Anthropological Approaches to the Study of Religion*. London: Routledge, 1–46.

Gell, Alfred (1998). *Art and Agency*. Oxford: Clarendon Press.

Gibson, James (1979). *In The Ecological Approach to Visual Perception*. Boston: Houghton Mifflin Harcourt.

Good, Byron J. (1993). *Medicine, Rationality and Experience: An Anthropological Perspective*. Cambridge: Cambridge University Press.

Hallowell, Alfred Irving (2002). Ojibwa Ontology, Behavior, and World View. In G. Harvey (Ed.), *Reading in Indigenous Religions*. London: Continuum, 18–49.

Hardon, A., and E. Moyer (2014). Medical technologies: Flows, frictions and new socialities. *Anthropology & Medicine* 21(2):107–112. DOI: 10.1080/1364 8470.2014.924300.

Heidegger, Martin (1971). *Poetry, Language, Thought*. Trans. Albert Hofstadter. New York: Harper & Row.

Herzfeld, Michael (1981). Meaning and morality: A semiotic approach to evil eye accusations in a Greek village. *American Ethnologist* 8(3): 560–574.

Ingold, Tim (2007). Materials against materiality. *Archaeological Dialogues* 14(1):1–16.

Ingold, Tim (2010a). Bringing Things Back to Life: Creative Entanglements in a World of Materials. ESRC National Centre for Research Methods. Working Paper Series 05/10 (2010). Accessed http://eprints.ncrm.ac.uk/1306/.

Ingold, Tim (2010b). The textility of making. *Cambridge Journal of Economics* 34(1):91–102.

Ingold, Tim and Gisli Palsson. (Eds.). (2013). *Biosocial Becomings: Integrating Social and Biological anthropology*. Cambridge. Cambridge University Press.

Justman, Stuart (2016). *The Nocebo Effect: Overdiagnosis and Its Costs*. New York: Springer.

Kandinsky, Wassily (2008 [1911]). *Concerning the Spiritual in Art*. Trans. Michael Sadler. Portland: The Floating Press.

Kleinman, Arthur (1980). *Patients and Healers in the Context of Culture: An Exploration of the Borderland between Anthropology, Medicine, and Psychiatry (Vol. 3)*. Berkeley: University of California Press.

Kleinman, Arthur and Peter Benson (2006). Anthropology in the clinic: The problem of cultural competency and how to fix it. *PLoS medicine* 3(10):e294.

Kleinman, Arthur, Leon Eisenberg and Byron Good (1978). Culture, illness, and care: Clinical lessons from anthropologic and cross-cultural research. *Annals of Internal Medicine* 88(2):251–258.

Latour, Bruno (1991). *We Have Never Been Modern*. Cambridge, MA: Harvard University Press.

Latour, Bruno (1993). *Aramis, or the Love of Technology*. Cambridge, MA: Harvard University Press.

Latour, Bruno (1999). *Pandora's Hope*. Cambridge, MA: Harvard University Press.

Lévi-Strauss, Claude (2000 [1949]). The Effectiveness of Symbols. In R Littlewood and S Dein (Eds.), *Cultural Psychiatry and Medical Anthropology: An Introduction and Reader*, 162.

Lewis-Fernández, Roberto, Neil Krishan Aggarwal, Sofie Bäärnhielm, Hans Rohlof, Laurence J. Kirmayer, Mitchell G. Weiss, Sushrut Jadhav et al. (2014). Culture and psychiatric evaluation: Operationalizing cultural formulation for DSM-5. *Psychiatry: Interpersonal and Biological Processes* 77(2):130–154.

Lipsedge, Maurice and Roland Littlewood (2005). *Aliens and Alienists: Ethnic Minorities and Psychiatry*. London: Routledge.

Littlewood, Roland (1992). Psychiatric diagnosis and racial bias: Empirical and interpretative approaches. *Social Science Medicine* 34(2):141–9.

Malinowski, Bronislow (1960 [1944]). *A Scientific Theory of Culture*. New York: Oxford University Press.

Martin, Emily (2006). The pharmaceutical person. *BioSocieties* 1:273–287.

Martin, Emily (2007). *Bipolar Expeditions: Mania and Depression in American Culture*. Princeton: Princeton University Press.

Mattingly, Cheryl (1994). The concept of therapeutic 'emplotment'. *Social Science & Medicine* 38(6):811–822.

Mertz, Elizabeth (2007). Semiotic anthropology. *Annual Review of Anthropology* 36:337–353.

Miller, Daniel (1997). *Material Cultures: Why Some Things Matter*. Chicago: University Chicago Press.

Moerman, Daniel E. (2002). *Meaning, Medicine, and the "Placebo Effect"* (Vol. 28). Cambridge: Cambridge University Press.

Mol, Annemarie (2002). *The Body Multiple: Ontology in Medical Practice*. London: Duke University Press.

Mol, Annemarie (2008). *The Logic of Care: Health and the Problem of Patient Choice*. London: Routledge.

Morgan, Lewis Henry (1877). *Ancient Society; or, Researches in the Lines of Human Progress from Savagery, through Barbarism to Civilisation*. New York; Henry Holt and Company.

Morphy, Howard (2009). Art as a mode of action: Some problems with Gell's Art and Agency. *Journal of Material Culture* 14(1):5–27.

Petryna, Adriana and Arthur Kleinman (2006). The Pharmaceutical Nexus. In A. Petryna, A. Lakoff and A. Kleinman (Eds.), *Global Pharmaceuticals: Ethics, Markets, Practices*. Durham, NC: Duke University Press, 1–32.

Pink, Sarah, J. Morgan, and A. Dainty (2014). The safe hand: Gels, water, gloves and the materiality of tactile knowing. *Journal of Material Culture* 19(4):425–42.

Požgain, I., Z. Požgain and D. Degmečić (2014). Placebo and nocebo effect: A mini-review. *Psychiatria Danubina* 26(2):100–107.

Propp, Vladimir (1968). *Morphology of the Folktale*. Trans. Laurence Scott; revised by Louis A. Wagner. Austin: University of Texas Press.

Rowlands, Michael (1983). Material culture studies at British Universities: University college London. *RAIN* (59):15–16.

Singer, Milton (1980). Signs of the self: An exploration in semiotic anthropology. *American Anthropologist* 82(3):485–507.

Singer, Merrill (1995). Beyond the ivory tower: Critical praxis in medical anthropology. *Medical Anthropology Quarterly* 9(1):80–106.

Sontag, Susan (1978). *Illness as Metaphor*. New York: Farrar, Straus and Giroux.

Sontag, Susan (1989). *AIDS and Its Metaphors*. New York: Farrar, Straus and Giroux.

Tilley, Chris (2007). Materiality in materials. *Archaeological Dialogues* 14(1):16–20.

Tropea, Savina (2012). 'Therapeutic emplotment': A new paradigm to explore the interaction between nurses and patients with a long-term illness. *Journal of Advanced Nursing* 68(4):939–947.

Turner, Victor W. (1964). An Ndembu doctor in practice. *Magic, Faith and Healing* 239:63.

Turner, Edith (1994). A Visible Spirit Form in Zambia. In D.E. Young and J. Goulet (Eds.), *Being Changed by Cross-Cultural Encounters: The Anthropology of Extraordinary Experience*. Peterborough: Broadview Press, 71–96.

Ucko, Peter (1969). Penis sheaths: A comparative study. *Proceedings of the RAI*: 24–67.

Were, Graeme (2013). On the materials of mats: Thinking through design in a Melanesian society. *Journal of the Royal Anthropological Institute* 19(3):581–599.

Whyte, S.R., S. Van der Geest and A. Hardon (2002). *Social Lives of Medicines*. Cambridge: Cambridge University Press.

Part I
Flesh and fluids

2 Of flesh and mesh

Time, materiality, and health in surgical recovery

Rebecca Lynch

Surgical interventions are not often the focus of medical anthropological projects and yet offer a way in which anthropologists might go 'beyond the body proper' (Farquhar and Lock 2007). This call for a different type of engagement with the body, alongside approaches that seek to include more material aspects of health and illness within an ethnographic study, challenge a division between the biological (or 'nature') as the site of investigation for medicine, and the social (or 'culture') as the point of interest for anthropology. Instead, this position argues that we can never be separated from the material world – our bodies and our health are both constituted of, and made through, the material.

A more traditional anthropological approach to surgery might focus on accounts of the experience of (in this case) the women undergoing surgery, decisions they have made around this, and attitudes towards their body and to medicine. It might also consider relations between medical professionals and how they interact with patients. By focusing on accounts and experiences and leaving everything within the skin as the domain of medicine, a distinction between the biological and the sociocultural is set up, with clinicians working in the domain of the former while the anthropological gaze is restricted to the latter. This dualist separation suggests that 'nature' and 'culture' can, and should, be examined separately, the boundaries between both clear and stable. Such a separation is directly challenged by work both within medical anthropology and in biomedicine, for example, on chronic conditions, epigenetics, and so-called lifestyle diseases. Through such examples, the social and biological cannot be so clearly drawn apart, and medical anthropologists increasingly look to include the materiality of the body in their work. Such an approach also challenges an acceptance of the body as a universal, uniform, and standard 'body proper.'

The body is obviously not a new focus within anthropology and has generated many different approaches, such as Durkheim's (1995 [1912]) split between higher socialised bodies and the physical body, Mary Douglas' (1973) natural bodies used as social analogies, and Foucauldian disciplinary bodies of governmentality (Foucault 1978, 1979). Embodiment approaches and the work of theorists such as Bourdieu (1984) and Shilling

(1993) point out that bodies are not born but made – by definition our bodies are cultural, not natural, as they are formed over time through experiences. More recently, Farquhar and Lock have drawn attention to the classic analysis of relationships between society and individuals drawn on by many social scientists. This requires what they term a 'proper' body through which to view the individuals who collectively make up society. The body proper is constructed in these analyses as 'a skin-bounded, rights-bearing, communicating, experience-collecting, biomechanical entity' (2007:2), a 'common sense' view of the body that does not allow for the diverse range of human experiences and relationships, and which separates mind from body, and subjective experience from material things. It also does not align with understandings within biomedicine, where medical interventions and implants, and understandings of ways our external and internal environments contribute to human health, challenge taken-for-granted ideas of biological separateness and the 'natural.' Instead Farquhar and Lock argue for 'an expanded anthropology of embodiment' (2007:12), the 'proper body' not sustainable with neither changing understandings of the make-up of the body, nor how cultural understandings and experiences, and the wider environment, affect it. The use of surgical mesh that becomes permanently attached to the interior of the body is one such example of troubling the boundaries of the body proper; it is less clear what is considered part of the 'natural' body and what is not. I draw on mesh not only to look at how we might think beyond the body proper through bodily integration, but also to consider when and where differences might be important and perhaps inevitable.

This chapter examines the use of mesh in surgery for stress urinary incontinence (SUI), an involuntary loss of urine during exertion, coughing, sneezing, or laughing, and pelvic organ prolapse (POP), the collapse of parts of the vagina. While leaking urine is connected to 'normal' ageing in men and women, this chapter examines the use of surgery offered by the UK NHS for women who experience a considerable impact on their quality of life from regular, and often significant, uncontrolled loss of urine. Both SUI and POP are understood to share a common cause: the weakening of muscular and connective tissues in the pelvic floor (Gigliobianco et al. 2015). This has been connected to not just ageing, but also obesity, pregnancy, and childbirth as well as menopause and genetic aspects of women themselves so that the range of women affected is broad. Physiotherapy is usually offered initially to address the problem; however, if symptoms persist, corrective surgery is seen as a more effective and longer lasting treatment. Synthetic mesh is commonly used during such surgery to reinforce pelvic floor repairs, and once inserted into the body it remains in place, integrating with and supporting the local tissues that form around it.

While surgeries for SUI and POP are recognised to be largely successful, both surgeries can cause complications such as pain, inflammation, and 'erosion' of tissues around the site of insertion. These complications differ between the surgeries, with greater problems with mesh erosion iden-tified for women undergoing POP repair than SUI surgery (Gigliobianco et al. 2015). Significantly, complications from the use of mesh are difficult to resolve: once mesh has started to integrate with flesh, it is not easy to remove. The last decade has seen a growth of reports of complications from POP mesh surgery, particularly drawing the attention of media and televi-sion in England in 2017. As such, non-success of such surgeries is also part the story of these interventions.

Taking up understandings that the material body is shaped by (and, indeed, shapes) society, what is more novel in newer approaches is the inclu-sion of material entities, including the non-human, within an ethnography. Part of acknowledging that society can never be separated from the mate-rial world is to see the material as part of society; a fuller ethnography also takes 'things' into account (Latour 2005). In fact, rather than starting with human-to-human relations and accounts, in the case of mesh surgery for pel-vic floor repair, we might instead focus on the nub of the issue: where flesh and mesh meet. To look only at surgical decision-making, or on patients' understandings and accounts of their experiences, misses the crucial aspect of surgery: its materiality.

Rather than focus on the (social) experiences of these women, I consider the materials themselves: the properties, affordances, and temporalities brought together during these surgeries and through which mesh and flesh integrate to create a new form within the human body. As Donna Hara-way (2008) suggests, part of becoming human is embracing and touching other things, and drawing on her work examining what is touched when humans and non-human are brought together may give us an alternative understanding of these surgeries, and perhaps a different way of viewing the body. Here, then, is the story of the integration of a material body and material technology, an action that folds in wider times and wider spaces. It is also a relationship forming over time, both the living organism of the body and a manufactured material implant in states of flux and change, nei-ther 'finished objects' but both 'becoming' into being (Ingold 2012). Because pelvic floor surgery is sometimes unsuccessful, it is also a story of how such a positive relationship may not develop, the failure as well as success of bringing together mesh and flesh.

Becoming material bodies

The turn moving 'beyond the body proper' in anthropology has also been undertaken in actor-network approaches and by philosophers of science and technology. Theorists such as Latour (2005), Hacking (1986), Hara-way (1991), Mol (2002), and Barad (2007) have been part of this mate-rialist movement, attending to ways in which bodies are made through practices and relations, not existing independently from these. Like Ingold, these scholars largely recognise bodies as a result of ongoing processes of becoming, the body 'a dynamic centre of unfolding activity, rather than a sink into which practices are sedimented' (Ingold 2012:439). Following Ingold (2010), Nading (2016) notes that health itself can be seen as constituted of and by things, non-living entities involved in its making and unmaking. Through these understandings, 'things' are integral to our well-being, part of dynamic processes that contribute to living. Things are also entities in process (Ingold 2010, 2012); humans and non-humans not only co-existing but generating conditions of possibility for their inter- and intra-action (Barad 2007; Ingold 2010). This, therefore, suggests a temporal dimension to these relationships and the potential for movement and flux; bodies and materials are not static, and neither are their connections to each other.

While Haraway's work on cyborgs has often been drawn on to consider the relationship between humans and technology and to deconstruct dualisms of self:other and natural:artificial (Haraway 1991), it is Haraway's concept of 'becoming with' that I wish to draw on here to look at the ongoing and temporally located relationships between mesh and flesh that these surgeries create. Developed through considering human relationships to other species, Haraway notes that the human body is made up of a range of bacteria, fungi, protists, and different microbiota and that becoming an adult human being is undertaken in company with these symbionts: 'To be one is always to *become with* many' (1991:4, emphasis in the original). Her work looks at the ways in which human and other lives (including her own and her dog's) are constituted in intra- and interaction with each other, co-shaping their existences through time. Her work advocates a multi-species ethnography and (as her cyborg work also proposes) challenges ideas of human exceptionalism, what she terms the 'Great Divide' between human and other. Like Latour, then, she suggests that the social is not exclusively made up of humans but also of other 'things' and our relations to these. For Haraway, becoming human involves relationships with non-humans, in and on our bodies as much as around them. Such an approach not only invites us to ask where the boundaries of the body might lie but also to attend to how we live with, and become through, such relations over our lifetimes (and beyond!) – how our bodies are 'becoming with' others.

Haraway's concept of 'becoming with' starts by asking 'what do I touch when I touch my dog?' (2008:3). To answer this question, Haraway demonstrates that she needs to consider the natural, social, cultural, political, and economic history of her dog's breed through colonialism alongside the natural, social, cultural, political, and economic properties shaping her interaction with her dog today. Haraway's approach, unlike Latour's flat ontology, is a critical social theory perspective of materiality through which we might bring together the multiple properties, practices, and discourses around the use of surgical mesh for pelvic organ collapse and urinary incontinence. If we follow Haraway's logic to look at non-human microorganisms as entities that are 'becoming with' the body, why not also include the material technologies embedded within it: the medical technologies and implants that also, in time, become part of the body? More significantly, perhaps, what new directions and questions might this approach open up when looking at surgical interventions?

The particular usefulness of this approach for looking at surgery results from two crucial aspects implicit in Haraway's question and its answer. First, that time is integral to becoming with: the properties of both sides being brought together while 'becoming with' is formed in time. Second, what Haraway terms 'touch across difference' reminds us that differences remain even as they encounter and shape the other. By attending to both time and difference, we might follow Haraway's line of questioning to ask, 'what is being touched when mesh is attached to flesh?' In so doing, we consider the natural, social, cultural, political, and economic history of both the mesh and the flesh as well as the time and space 'folded' into these (Latour 2002). As such, we might think of bodies and medical materials not only in the process of becoming as Ingold suggests, but also as 'becoming with.' Furthermore, in the context of pelvic floor surgery, we may also acknowledge 'failing to become with,' instances where touching does not bring integration and positive health outcomes, but instead stubborn difference and resulting iatrogenesis (harm caused by biomedical diagnosis or therapeutic intervention).

Touching mesh and flesh

Latour (2002) and others have drawn on Serres' work to suggest that pasts are enfolded in objects. As Latour (2002) illustrates with his workbench hammer, technologies enfold heterogenous temporalities and spaces: the antiquity of the planet within the moulded mineral hammerhead, the age of the oak in the handle, the year it was created through factory production as well as the different locations of forest, mine, factory, sales van, and workshop. But, he suggests, this is not enough. The actor, the other entities involved (such as nails), and action of the hammer are also folded in, the different forms hammers have taken in different places and the possibilities of use suggesting an additional focus on the affordances of the technology. I focus here on how temporalities and properties and affordances enfolded in mesh technology and the flesh onto which it is placed enable 'becoming with,' so that body and implant continue to work together.

Mesh

A range of medical devices has been implanted in people for many decades, including artificial knees and hips, and metallic support for bones. These devices are intended to stay within the body and become part of it, as is also the case with mesh technologies. Mesh becomes integrated into the area of the body it is used on, forming a permanent attachment that reinforces the tissue it is fixed to. The use of mesh to support prolapsed organs and the urethra requires the recognition of particular symptoms being resolved through such supportive interventions: that urinary incontinence is, for example, a particular kind of problem with a particular kind of solution. In this case, it was Ulmsten and Petros' 'integral theory of urinary incontinence' (Petros and Ulmsten 1990; Ulmsten and Petros 1993) that initiated the development of these surgeries. Following the success of mesh slings implanted under the middle of the urethra to support it, mesh was later introduced in pelvic organ prolapse repair.

Transvaginal mesh (for POP) and mid-urethral slings (for SUI) are made of polypropylene, the same material used for repairs of hernias and for sutures. Polypropylene was made initially in 1954, with its usefulness for mesh hernia repair understood by herniologist Francis C. Usher in 1962, partly due to its ability to be autoclaved (sterilised using steam) (Kelly et al. 2017). Polypropylene mesh has undergone intensive testing for its use on hernias, where there is good evidence of effective outcomes (Gigliobianco et al. 2015). However, its approval for POP and SUI was not based on long-term supportive data. Instead, a 'grandfather clause' where a new material was permitted based on its similarity to its use elsewhere (i.e. in hernias) allowed its introduction for use in other places in the body. This policy suggests that it is the material composition and physical properties of the technology that are of most concern in relation to the insertion of biomaterials in the body, rather than where in the body the technology is being used. Through this argument, mesh technology is seen as somewhat neutral, acting the same way in one part of the body as in another. It assumes that 'flesh' and 'mesh' relate to each other in broadly the same way, no matter which flesh and which mesh are being brought together.

At the level of design, however, mesh appears less neutral. While meshes for the treatment of stress incontinence and vaginal prolapse have similarities, they are configured differently for these different interventions (Kelly et al. 2017), the affordances of different mesh configurations bringing different possibilities into being. Mesh is classified into four groups depending on pore size, with larger sized pores allowing for 'superior tissue integration,' as collagen can better form across them. As well as promoting integration, pore size also has a role in preventing bacterial infection. Pathogens are smaller than the cells involved in the body's immune response; as such, mesh pores that allow pathogens but no immune response cells to penetrate could mean that bacteria would be able to remain on the mesh unchallenged (Kelly et al. 2017). The weight of the mesh is also important. The heavier the mesh, the greater the stiffening of tissue and the inability of the tissue to contract, a particular issue when attached to the walls of the vagina. However, mesh that is too light may not be suitable for handling, as the mesh is folded when it is inserted. Any material used needs to be robust enough to withstand surgical handling and insertion as well as provide flexible support within the body. Mesh design demonstrates that in reinforcing flesh, mesh also needs to be able to do other work: supporting collagen growth, allowing immune response to bacteria, sustaining manipulation during surgery, and so on. Mesh is thus active in repairing flesh in a number of different ways.

There are also different entry points to surgical insertion and different procedures used in such instances to attach the mesh to different places. These are associated with different degrees of success; for example, there is an increased risk of infection associated with vaginal insertion (Kelly et al. 2017). While a similar grade of mesh is used in different pelvic organ surgeries, as it is configured differently for different surgeries, interventions for SUI and POP are not singular but take multiple forms, allowing for differences between patients and surgeons. While this might, again, at the surface level, imply that mesh is a neutral material but patients and surgeries are different, we might instead suggest that different practices make different mesh (Mol 2002). Different sites and methods of insertion therefore make the affordances of mesh as variable as the affordances of flesh.

Flesh

One of the inevitable impacts of inserting mesh into the body is that it triggers a 'foreign body response' (Brown and Finch 2010). This causes inflammation and pain, and yet is also desirable to some extent. Inflammation is an important and complex process that not only clears the wound of abnormal cells and debris but also enables the remodelling and regeneration of tissue (Moalli et al. 2014). Some degree of response in the flesh is helpful, therefore, whereas too much becomes detrimental. The degree of response can alter depending on where in the body the mesh is implanted – in other words, which flesh is involved. For example, a number of studies have found that mesh used in the vaginal area is more susceptible to complications and a greater foreign body response than when mesh is inserted into the abdomen (Kelly et al. 2017). Individual bodily anatomy and immune systems also affect the body's response: obese bodies, older bodies, bodies with other illnesses, and those that have suffered trauma during parturition are viewed as being more problematic. If the inserted material is recognised as non-self and isolated from the body, it is not integrated with surrounding tissue. The mesh may not be sufficiently attached, tissues around the implant eroded through bacterial infection, or failure of flesh and mesh to integrate in particular areas. The affordances not only of different flesh in the body but also different bodies allow 'becoming with' mesh in different ways.

That these bodies are presented for surgery in the first place is also understood to rely on patient difference. Guidelines recommend that surgeons choosing between different surgical procedures should weigh up the potential risks and 'adverse events' of such interventions against the goals and wishes of the patients, the weighting of particular complications potentially differing not only between surgeon and patient but also between patients. Decisions might be whether 'objective cure' of urinary incontinence is more important than sexual function following surgery, for example (Schimpf et al. 2014). Which does the patient value more? This suggests a difference not only in the physical bodies of patients therefore, but also in their values and experiences. Temporalities are enfolded in the body and body parts, creating particular affordances of the flesh: women's experiences, age, lifestyle, childbearing, anatomy, and immune system all contribute to the degree of the problem and the possibility of change.

Also enfolded within flesh are the material and structural understandings of the cause of urinary incontinence, the availability of surgeries to intervene, and a wider movement from woman needing to put up with leaking to being able to discuss and have such symptoms addressed. Neither the patient nor the patient body are singular and standard, and each brings different surgeries and surgical outcomes into possibility. Surgical expertise based on training and experience are also considered to be key factors in the outcomes of pelvic floor procedures (Gigliobianco et al. 2015); such guidelines assume a degree of difference in surgeons as well as patients. It should be noted too that polypropylene mid-urethral slings are not the only treatment for SUI, and there is disagreement within urogynaecology around the use of tests to diagnose SUI before surgery (Lee and Zimmerman 2016). Biomedicine is not monolithic, and surgeons too are not a singular whole.

An approach focusing on patients' values and experiences, and perhaps also the experiences and decision-making of surgeons, not only reinforces a nature:culture divide but also misses the ways in which surgical outcomes are embedded in material possibilities. The temporalities, properties, and affordances of both mesh and flesh suggest the many complex relationships from which becoming with is possible including the sheer diversity present in both mesh and flesh. There is no one nature and one culture at stake here. Embodied experiences of childbirth, ageing, and (in the case of surgeons) undertaking surgery itself, the history and development of mesh of a particular size and shape, the location of surgical intervention and mode of insertion, the body's physicality, and the body's immune response are all relevant and the success of the surgery is distributed across these aspects. This is not the result of pure relationally but rather what Ingold (2012) terms 'webs of life.' Rather than suggesting a standardised and singular surgery on a singular body proper, a positive outcome needs to occur *despite* such different bodies and different surgeries. Becoming with does not rely on sameness or complete merger, therefore, but of retaining and working with difference.

Mesh-flesh

Two different materials with different properties, affordances, and temporalities enfolded within them are brought together through surgery to form a new integrated material: mesh-flesh. It is the successful creation of mesh-flesh that will support portions of the woman's internal structure by becoming part of her body, a meshing that will allow for 'normal' functioning.

Integration does not occur immediately in surgery, however; this new material develops over time. Rather than a sole touching and co-existence of flesh and mesh, a constantly developing process is required that the surgery itself merely instigates. This highlights two crucial coalescences of time in relation to the fusing of mesh-flesh: the surgical event and recovery after surgery. While there is clearly a relationship between the two (how the mesh is put in, how the surgery is carried out including the use of instruments and their cleanliness, for example), the many months, and sometimes years, of bodily repair that follow surgery are when the process of developing mesh-flesh takes place. Recovery takes time; indeed, recovery is time. As Ingold notes, 'Materials are not *in* time: they are the stuff of time itself' (2012:439).

These are, of course, not the only changes taking place within the body. The body is always in a state of repair and flux. Cells die and are replaced, the immune system works to identify and neutralise pathogens and cancer cells, nutrients are absorbed through the gut, hormones are released, blood flows, the body is never static. These go on alongside, and contribute to, the integration of flesh and mesh. Over time, these result in longer term bodily changes. We age, become fat, build immunity, and lose flexibility, skin elasticity, and bone density. The mesh becomes part of the body. Ingold's (2012) proposition that the body is dynamic and always in a state of becoming not only is a material observation but also suggests a movement forward in time that alters: the body is always in process, and that changes us. We are neither static, nor returning to homeostasis (Canguilhem 1989 [1978]); we are not the person we were yesterday. As part of the body changing over time, the boundaries between self and non-self are always being negotiated, including within the body itself.

Surgical recovery is 'successful' if mesh and flesh come together in a way that improves a woman's health and experiences. 'Becoming with' relies on a positive relationship, and 'health' here relies on a particular type of integration to occur, demonstrable on some occasions and not on others. A failure to sufficiently integrate can cause damage, disease, distress. Bodies are not standard, and mesh is not inert: they both carry different temporalities and practices, and it is perhaps not surprising that sometimes different types of integration occur. Failing to become with involves a drawing away. Both mesh and flesh may fail to integrate with the wider body and become foreign objects within it, causing damage rather than contributing to the health of its wider whole. Their difference is unable to be integrated and becomes intolerable.

Even in cases of successful becoming with, we might ask when the integration is complete. Both flesh and mesh continue to change and become more and more interwoven over time, but this is merely an issue of scale. The closer one looks, a point at which they remain separate becomes visible. At the cellular level, mesh never becomes flesh. Similarities and differences between what is 'flesh' and what 'mesh' are, therefore, determined not only over time, but also by scale. At what point might we suggest there is no difference? Such a separation between the two is problematic only when these do not fully work together. Lack of separation is also an issue as partially integrated mesh-flesh cannot be pulled apart and so moved or extracted from the body. To try to remove this would cause greater damage than leaving failing mesh-flesh in place. Mesh-flesh remains hyphenated, therefore, always two things as well as being one. Difference is retained, even at the optimal level of integration.

Recovery and health

When we consider the use of synthetic surgical mesh as a method of repairing or supporting damaged tissue such as supporting the vaginal wall following prolapse, to exclude the material interaction between mesh and flesh excludes the key issue. A focus on the material, however, also allows us to see the surgery and the body in a different way. The meeting points between flesh and mesh are not about the problems of a 'natural' body encountering a 'synthetic' material, but how two things work alongside each other, how they are becoming with. This is not dissimilar from other components in the body; indeed, health results from just such an integrated difference, and mesh is, therefore, similar in this way to any other part of the body.

No body is a single entity but is made up of different elements that integrate with each other, working together but not merging. Blood, for example, passes around bodily organs but does not become them. Blood itself is not singular: it includes red blood cells, white blood cells (leukocytes), platelets, water, and serum (which itself contains antibodies, anti-microbial proteins, etc.). Even at the level of the cell, there is a compartmentalisation of the nucleus, mitochondria, Golgi, and ribosomes. Depending on scale, these are part of the same thing or separate entities: like mesh-flesh, the body is at once one entity and many different things at the same time. Such differences are important for becoming with, a story of relatedness and incorporation. Mesh-flesh is not about becoming the same thing but rather aligning together over time again, much like the rest of the body. The division between 'natural' and 'artificial' materials in the body is, therefore, difficult to locate: at one scale, the same and at another, quite different.

As with the problems of correcting complications caused by mesh, we might consider whether it is detrimental to the whole to pull these materials apart. A focus on mesh-flesh suggests that the body is always about distinction *as well as* integration. Furthermore, this is a continual incorporation and integration of difference, never complete as the body creates new cells and gets rid of others; it circulates, metabolises, excretes. The body is always literally becoming. Health is distributed across, but also relies on such processes: processes that take place over time and change our bodies in doing so. Recovery is not, therefore, to return to what one once was but rather to be changed, and to be able to continue to change: the body becoming with.

Differences are inherent in the properties and affordances of bodies, and in the surgical interventions in which they are involved. Surgeries bring together new combinations of these and start new relationships between entities inserted or removed, initiating new temporalities and processes of change, and setting up the conditions of possibility for incorporation of difference over time. Once the conditions of possibility for the body's becoming are in place, integration and difference depends on scale as well as time. Recovery is dependent on these factors coming together.

Material properties and affordances 'do' things, therefore: they bring various possibilities into being, including if we scale up, improvements to everyday life. Attending to the properties and affordances of the material, the normative assumptions within their design, manufacture, and use, as well as the changes they initiate over time and at particular scales, allows us to bring together material changes within cells and tissues with individual experiences and with wider socio-cultural ideals and understandings. The turn to materiality brings a 'zooming in' through which difference and integration at different scales in the body is visible, but if we attend to what else in enfolded within the material, it may also allow us to 'zoom out,' even to helping us think through ways in which we might examine the body in medical anthropology.

As noted earlier, being human involves becoming with many (Haraway 2008). Maintaining difference at different scales can be productive as well as inevitable. Understanding that the body is neither singular nor static, and its boundaries are always up for negotiation, we might take these arguments further to recognise how medical anthropological approaches to the body are likewise plural, dynamic, and changing, and not clearly bounded. Rather than separate, exclude, or neatly demarcate one approach from another, we might instead think about ways, places, scales, and times in which we might integrate or keep as different these various approaches. How might we pull together material approaches to the body with Douglas' (1973) symbolic 'natural' bodies, for example, and what might this tell us in doing so? What novel directions and questions are raised by attending to time in the body in relation both to biological processes and bodily experiences? How might we best bring together the complexities of bodies at different scales so that individual biologies can also be related to global health policy? Such questions appear increasingly salient as anthropologists conduct ethnographies not only of laboratories but also of multinationals, health and the body appearing as different things at these different scales (Yates-Doerr 2015). If a more in-depth ethnography also involves things, and if fieldsites could potentially be exponential, defining the foci of ethnography might also depend on how to speak across scales and incorporate difference. Mesh, flesh, and mesh-flesh in this case provide the perfect analogies – at some points integration occurs where elsewhere difference is inevitable, while tearing apart integrated material may be detrimental to the whole. As with the insertion of surgical mesh too, bringing together different approaches to the body in medical anthropology might initially involve agitation and inflammation; however, this is a necessary part of fuller integration.

In line with this argument, therefore, is not a call to abandon all previous anthropological approaches to the body but to use material aspects to think through these more broadly, bringing together different pieces and raising new questions. Here, I have drawn attention to where the boundaries of our bodies might lie, how we live with and become through relations with non-humans, and how becoming with occurs despite and across difference involving distinction as well as integration. Using the idea that a healthy body is one that is able to tolerate and integrate difference, and can continue to become with in correspondence with different elements over time, may help us move from a focus on ill bodies to bodies in health and perhaps cause us to ask, what is a body in the first place?

Acknowledgements

Many thanks to Simon Cohn for his comments in the development of this chapter. The chapter was written while employed on the National Institute of Health Research project 'Surgical Care for Female Urinary Incontinence' (NIHR HS&DR 14/70/162). I am grateful for the support of the wider project team at LSHTM, led by Prof. Jan van der Meulen.

References

Barad, K. (2007). *Meeting the Universe Halfway: Quantum Physics and the Entanglement of Matter and Meaning*. Durham: Duke University Press.

Bourdieu, P. (1984). *Distinction: A Social Critique of the Judgment of Taste*. London: Routledge.

Brown, C.N. and J.G. Finch (2010). Which mesh for hernia repair? *Annals of the Royal College of Surgeons of England* 92(4):272–278.

Canguilhem, G. (1989). *The Normal and the Pathological*. Reprint of 1978 issue. New York: Zone Books.

Douglas, M. (1973). *Natural Symbols. Explorations in Cosmology*. Second edition. London: Barrie and Jenkins Ltd.

Durkheim, E. (1995 [1912]). *The Elementary Forms of the Religious Life*. Trans. Karen E. Fields. New York: Free Press.

Farquhar, J. and M. Lock (2007). Introduction. In M. Lock and J. Farquhar (Eds.), *Beyond the Body Proper: Reading the Anthropology of Material Life*. Durham and London: Duke University Press.

Foucault, M. (1978). *The History of Sexuality*, Vol. 1. New York: Pantheon Books.

Foucault, M. (1979). *Discipline and Punish: The Birth of the Prison*. New York: Vintage.

Gigliobianco, G., S.R. Regueros, N.J. Osman, J. Bissoli, A.J. Bullock, C.R. Chapple and S. MacNeil (2015). Biomaterials for pelvic floor reconstructive surgery: How can we do better? *BioMed Research International* 2015 Article ID 968087, 20 pages. DOI: 10.1155/2015/968087.

Hacking, I. (1986). Making up People. In T.C. Heller, M. Sosna, and D.E. Wellbery (Eds.), *Reconstructing Individualism: Autonomy, Individuality, and the Self in Western Thought*. Stanford: Stanford University Press, 222–236.

Haraway, D. (1991). *Simians, Cyborgs, and Women: The Reinvention of Nature*. London: Free Association Books.

Haraway, D. (2008). *When Species Meet*. Minneapolis: University of Minnesota Press.

Ingold, T. (2010). Bringing things to life: Creative entanglements in a world of materials. *Realities Working Paper Series No.15*. Manchester UK: Economic and Social Research Council.

Ingold, T. (2012). Toward an ecology of materials. *Annual Review of Anthropology* 41:427–442.

Kelly, M., K. Macdougall, O. Olabisi, and N. McGuire (2017). In vivo response to polypropylene following implantation in animal models: A review of biocompatibility. *International Urogynecology Journal* 28(2):171–180.

Latour, B. (2002). Morality and technology: The end of the means. *Theory, Culture & Society* 19:247–260.

Latour, B. (2005). *Reassembling the Social: An Introduction to Actor-Network-Theory*. Oxford: Oxford University Press.

Lee, D. and P.E. Zimmerman (2016). Evaluation of stress urinary incontinence: State-of-the-art review. *European Medical Journal* 1(3):103–110.

Moalli, P., B. Brown, M. T. F. Reitman, and C. W. Nager (2014). Polypropylene mesh: Evidence for lack of carcinogenicity. *International Urogynecology Journal* 25(5):573–576.

Mol, A. (2002). *The Body Multiple: Ontology in Medical Practice*. Durham & London: Duke University Press.

Nading, A. (2016). Local biologies, leaky things, and the chemical infrastructure of global health. *Medical Anthropology* 36(2):141–156.

Petros P. and U. Ulmsten (1990). An integral theory of female urinary incontinence. *Acta Obstetricia et Gynaecologica Scandinavica* 69(Suppl.153):1–79.

Schimpf, M.O., D.D. Rahn, T.L. Wheeler, M. Patel, A.B. White, F.J. Orejuela, S.A. El-Nashar, R.U. Margulies, J.L. Gleason, S.O. Aschkenazi, M.M. Mamik, R.M. Ward, E.M. Balk, V.W. Sung, for the Society of Gynecologic Surgeons Systematic Review Group (2014). Sling surgery for stress urinary incontinence in women: A systematic review and metaanalysis. *American Journal of Obstetrics & Gynecology* 211(1):71e1–71e27.

Shilling, C. (1993). *The Body and Social Theory*. London: Sage.

Ulmsten, U. and P. Petros (1993). An integral theory and its method for the diagnosis and treatment of female urinary incontinence. *Scandinavian Journal of Urology and Nephrology* Supp. 153.

Yates-Doerr, E. (2015). Intervals of confidence: Uncertain accounts of global hunger. *Biosocieties* 10(2):229–246.

3   From attitudes to materialities
Understanding bowel control for colorectal cancer patients in London

Ignacia Arteaga

An unproblematic surgical procedure

Planned bowel surgery to resect a malignant tumour requires patients to physically, emotionally, and intellectually prepare for it. A surgeon met Jay, a British man in his thirties of Indian background affected with stage III rectal cancer, to explain the procedure. He would undergo a *colectomy*, that is, the 'en bloc resection' of a large area of the large intestine where the tumour sits, which includes its vascular and lymphatic structures and cancer-free tissue margins. Because of the site and stage of his cancer, measured via scans and colonoscopies at the moment of diagnosis, the multidisciplinary team that oversees patients' treatments suggested that Jay should have a permanent *colostomy* – that is, the diversion of the bowel towards a surgical opening on the abdominal wall where the upper end of the bowel is sewn, forming a stoma. Plastic surgery would then be performed to close his excised rectum and anus. Three defining aspects of the body – function, sensation, and image – would permanently change after the stoma formation.

After discussing with the surgeon the main risks of the procedure and fertility preservation options, Jay was given homework to do. He was invited to meet a former patient treated by the same surgeon for the same condition. This way, Jay could see first-hand how someone with a colostomy could get on with life and understand that, regardless of how gruesome the stoma formation might initially feel, people manage to adapt to it over time. Jay was also invited to talk with a bowel cancer specialist nurse to find out what to expect from his bowel function after surgery and to find out how to look after his stoma. Jay's faecal waste was to be collected in a plastic pouch attached to the left lower side of his abdomen. However, as a large part of the bowel had been resected, bowel outputs would change consistency considerably towards more liquid states. 'The large intestine is the part of the body that drinks water for us,' the stoma nurse explained to another patient I was following. That means that without big sections of the large bowel, water and mineral absorption processes that started in the small intestine cannot be completed before they are evacuated. A week before surgery, Jay underwent a clinical pre-assessment, in which a nurse interviewed him to determine his physical and psychological fitness for surgery.

Three days before surgery, Jay received a 'bowel preparation package' by post, containing laxative sachets to consume over a few days, on top of the requirement to drastically eliminate his fibre intake before surgery. The aim was to get his intestines as clean and empty as possible in order to make things easier for the surgeons, and to minimise the risk of infection from faecal matter soiling the peritoneum during surgery. As he was undergoing 'elective' (pre-booked), rather than emergency, surgery to repair an obstructed or perforated intestine, the surgeons were able to use a procedure called the 'key-hole technique.' Instead of a long abdominal cut, this procedure consists of a series of small incisions through which surgical instruments such as miniature cameras and lanterns can be inserted. Everything went according to plan, and Jay recovered in hospital until he could eat a diet of soft foods and pass faecal waste without complications or debilitating pain. Just a few hours after he had fully awoken from the general anaesthetics, a stoma nurse visited him in the ward to teach him how to clean his stoma in practice. His concentration was low and his mind still foggy, but he had all his life to become acquainted with his new body part, and to improve his cleaning technique.

Four years after the first cancer diagnosis, three surgeries, a course of chemotherapy and fertility treatment, Jay is hitting his forties. He is the father of a young boy, the landlord of a flat in London, and the founder of his own estates company. Jay's ability to get to this point is not only because of his pragmatic attitude and resolution, the loving support of his wife and father, and comfortable finances. He was also, in some regards, lucky – having access to the benefits of modern surgery as a techno-scientific achievement. Surgical colectomy has been practised since 1776, but it became a safe procedure only when anatomical knowledge was coupled with effective antiseptic surgical techniques at the beginning of the twentieth century (Cromar 1968). Moreover, Jay benefitted from a further technological innovation that took place in 1991 when the laparoscope was created to replace direct contact between surgeon's hands and patients' viscera (Jacobs et al. 1991). Jay's successful experience of laparoscopic surgery confirmed the shorter recovery period it affords in comparison to laparotomy (open surgery). The procedure also minimises post-surgical pain and infection risk (Kuhry et al. 2008).

The current practice of oncological care for intestinal cancer in London is based on colectomies with or without colostomies, standing as the most effective treatment with curative intent for eligible[1] bowel cancer patients

---

1 Patient fitness for surgery, in consideration to frailty and co-morbidities, is analysed in conjunction with the progression stage with which the tumour is labelled during diagnosis to assess prognosis. Cancer stages are retrieved from imaging techniques and histological samples with standard labelling techniques that include three main components: size of the tumour, nodule involvement, and degree of metastasis (or whether the cancer has spread to other organs). Stages range from stage 0 to stage IV, which are then used to discern the appropriate clinical management of the condition, including the decision for surgery.

(NICE 2011). Complete surgical excision of the cancer growth offers the possibility to some people affected by colorectal cancer to eradicate the disease from their lives. During 17 months of ethnographic field research on everyday experiences of colorectal cancer treatments in London, I quickly realised how significant surgery was for all my research participants. Surgical findings and outcomes structure consecutive clinical procedures, depending on histological analysis of the tissue, the visual corroboration of the tumour spread (including extra-mural invasion and number of lymph nodes involved), and the success in resecting the mass with margins free of mutated cells. Surgery was also vividly narrated by many patients as the single cause for their survival from cancer, notwithstanding the complications they might have endured on the way. Hence, the creation of the artificial anus on one side of the abdominal wall is, from the patients' point of view, one of the most important features of their treatment experience.

It takes considerable time for the human body to 're-learn' the peristaltic rhythms of the bowel after surgery. As a consequence of the resection, patients like Jay must cope with increased bowel motility. But the stoma does not have a sphincter, and without it, defecation occurs without Jay's control. Even for patients who did not need a stoma after the surgical resection (i.e. had a colectomy without colostomy), diarrhoea is a debilitating side effect of cancer treatments. It requires people to deal with a metabolic rhythm and a material messiness that all colorectal cancer patients experience but is especially highlighted if their intestines become obstructed. Unlike scholarship highlighting the difficulty for people with stomas to reconstruct their self-image after surgery in order to socially reintegrate (Tao et al. 2014; Thorpe et al. 2009) as the main source of stress post-surgery, my ethnography highlights the importance of its precondition. The management of high-output stomas during cancer treatment in order to regain bowel control is, therefore, an essential task for my research participants. The challenge, I would like to argue, relates to our understanding of what diverted bowels and ostomy pouches afford the person to do, analysing the material conditions that enable cancer patients to be in control of their bowel outputs. The practice of managing bowel motility makes it possible to present an anatomically different body to oneself and to the world. The psycho-social understanding of adjustment, in this vein, could be complemented with an analysis of what happens before the attitudes with which a person relates to his or her stoma, incorporating the multiple materialities at play.

In understanding the practices and materials through which people with stomas are able to carry on with their everyday routines, I wish to depart from symbolic analyses of matters out of place that have permeated anthropological analysis of (in)continence and defecation practices (Douglas 2003; Lea 2001; Lawton 1998; Manderson 2005; van der Geest 2007). Undoubtedly, the symbolic aspects that connote matters out of place are relevant to understand the practices that my interlocutors develop to conceal the stoma and its 'accidents' from others. Yet I would like to argue that symbolic approaches to 'dirt' miss the perspectives of people with stomas, and make the experience of incontinence something deviant. Writing in the third perspective obscures the struggle of those who are actually breaching the symbolic boundary. An exclusive consideration of the 'generalised other's' view of dirt, namely, the 'other' with a normative body, the 'other' that acts according to what is desirable, re-victimises the person who suffers from faecal incontinence. In doing so, symbolic analyses about social constructs of 'dirt' do not only reproduce a sanitised anthropological practice (Loudon 1975), but also such scholarship neglects to recognise the ways in which the production of such distinctions requires symmetry in the analysis. 'Matter out of place' is not only a construct imposed on 'dirty' individuals by the 'pure,' but also negotiated and informed by those who are made subject to this symbolic category.

Instead of focusing on the symbolic aspects of living with stomas, this chapter takes seriously the material interface that makes waste management possible for my research participants. I would like to offer an alternative, de-normativising view of stoma care that foregrounds the materiality of the body in its engagement with the physical and social surroundings. Following Tilley (2007), I understand materiality as not only incorporating the world of 'brute' objects that are oblivious to human actions (such as a standard ostomy pouch), but also the 'processual significance' of those materials and its properties for the 'socio-political relationships' between people. Tilley proposes a movement away from consideration of the raw materials towards its social significance, for [. . . materials are] implicated in people's experiences of the world, 'providing affordances for thought and action' (2007:17–19). Following this approach, I would like to examine the material properties of intestines at their interface with ostomy bags in order to tease out the modes through which material adjustment (dis)enable my research participants in their quest for achieving normal routines. Going beyond the body as representation to understand how it is made to work in practice, I suggest that the ability to manage the stoma lies in great part on the privilege of access to material devices and infrastructures tightly related to the social and economic support available to the person. Through the analysis of three different ethnographic cases, this chapter sheds light on two related questions: how do material techniques and infrastructures afford liveable stoma management routines? And, how do those practices afford different emotional states for the person with a body-with-stoma? A fine-tuned understanding of both questions might help to demystify the process through which clinical professionals assess people's 'adjustment' to stoma formations, offering instead a materialist understanding of behaviour change.

Colostomies and accidents

When I met Elizabeth, she was sitting in a wheelchair, speaking in Spanish with her sister, while she was waiting for her appointment with the medical oncologist. It was her sixth cycle of chemotherapy after bowel surgery. In a loud tone of voice that disturbed the constrained atmosphere of the clinic, she consented to participate in my research and told me the beginning of her cancer journey. She explained the process to me as follows: the tumour in her bowel was resected only at the third surgical attempt. During the first surgery, Elizabeth suffered a severe reaction to the anaesthesia which caused life-threatening breathing difficulties, known as *anaphylaxis*. During the second surgery, exactly on month after the first attempt, she haemorrhaged while undergoing laparoscopic surgery. This constituted a second medical emergency that required the surgeons to cut her abdominal area open to find and stop the internal bleeding. The surgical team induced her into a coma, and provided blood transfusions to stabilise her. She stayed four days in the intensive care unit until the surgeons were able to resume the operation with a third attempt. A stoma was created to facilitate an optimum recovery, which caused her a great shock. In her words:

> *The stoma nurse came every day to the ward to help me with the stoma. In the beginning I did not want to know about it, I did not want to see it. It was horrendous, much bigger! I cried a lot, but the nurse comforted me saying that it would get better, that I would learn how to manage it. She taught me and my children how it works, so they could support me.*

> (Elizabeth, age between 50–60 years)

Despite the fright that Elizabeth's children felt, their mother no longer had tumours in her bowel. With a clear histological margin around the area, the surgery had been successful in eradicating the cancer. Elizabeth was emphatic in showing her appreciation for the surgeon's power. Even though she went through severe complications, developing later a voluminous abdominal hernia around the site of the stoma, and long-standing pain in her legs because of nerve damage, she was quick to tell everyone that 'Dr O saved my life twice' – first by managing the anaphylaxis, and second by completely resecting her tumour. I followed her through seven out of 12 chemotherapy cycles, a partial liver resection, and the reversal of her colostomy after a year from initial surgery. After multiple cases of deep wound infections after every intestinal surgery, she is now recovering at home. She is working to feel physically and emotionally fit to go back to work in the catering industry where her boss waits for her arrival. Before the stoma reversal, she did not feel able to go to work, due to the possibility of leakages from her stoma.

Bowel and waste 'accidents,' the emic concept for leakages, are a common and powerful experience during treatment. Sitting in a coffee shop near the hospital together with her children and a close friend, Elizabeth and I were celebrating that she had received the twelfth and last cycle of chemotherapy after two surgical operations. Going through follow-up plans, she seamlessly started a story about an accident she suffered because of her stoma, with her children already laughing about it. Elizabeth, instead, wanted to convey her frustration to me:

> *It was the Saturday after chemotherapy [and I had diarrhoea]. I went to celebrate [my daughter] Sandra's birthday to a Chinese restaurant with my family. The stoma bag blew up while sitting on the table. I got the tablecloth dirty together with all my clothes. I went to the toilets area, crying from embarrassment, until one became available. I used wipes to clean myself and took off one of the t-shirts I was wearing too. Once in the bus back home, I was smelling the stinky odour of my faeces again, but my son-in-law convinced me that it was only my mind playing games with me, that he could only smell the lotion I used after changing the bag. Yet Sandra realised that it was not a mind game. The bag was leaking again, the diarrhoea was like water, non-stop [Elizabeth exclaims in the middle of the coffee shop while her children and friend openly laugh]. As soon as we got home, I went to the shower, taking everything off once I was inside the shower.*

Although her children did not think of this accident as a serious matter of concern, for it was not the first or last time it would happen to her, Elizabeth was certainly worried. I tried to calm her down and repeated what I had learned from the specialist nurses and oncologists: 'After chemo, you will not have so much diarrhoea, so it will become more controllable,' I said. She instead replied to me that she is afraid to go back to work. 'Just thinking in the probability of the accident, even if it is less likely [after chemo] makes me panic.' Joseph, her son, supported her: 'It is about the possibility, even if the probability is low.' Defecation can be considered as a cleansing ritual that is essential for any living organism. Yet it seems that its power is conferred only to those who are in control of the act, who can manage the spatio-temporality of its occurrence (Lea 2001). What happens when individuals have no control of their sphincters anymore? I am interested in exploring the productivity of accidents to understand how people with stomas cope with its threat and re-make their bodies through ordinary practices of care. In the next section, I will describe the material properties of the ostomy bag, the single most important material device to achieve bowel continence.

The humble but powerful pouch

Resonating with a long history of public stigmatisation against colostomies because of their 'disgusting consequences' until the twentieth century (Cromar 1968), Elizabeth's account of her stoma, and the fear to have accidents, points to the importance of nicely fitting ostomy bags to secure an emotional state that enables people with stoma to go on with their lives. Faecal incontinence was an issue professionally taken up by the incipient training of specialist stoma nurses in the UK back in 1980 (Lewis 1999). Before, people with stomas relied on cotton pads and collecting devices made of tin and silver to stop faecal leakage. Only in 1940 did people with faecal incontinence start using a washable rubber bag tied to the body with strings. While these bags absorbed unpleasant smells, they also caused intestinal prolapses (protrusion of the bowel through the stoma) and painful excoriation of the area. The solution appeared when plastic started to be industrially manufactured and used for stoma care in 1960, and people could resort to disposable pouches. That invention was coupled with the creation of protective barriers for the skin to prevent dermatitis, and hypo-allergenic adhesives originally invented for dentistry were repurposed as care for the skin (Lewis 1999).

While people undergoing colostomies might recover their bowel habits they practised before surgery, chemotherapy abruptly increases bowel motility and accidents happen with frequency. Clinical professionals recommend that their patients undergoing chemotherapy refrain from intestinal irrigation techniques to manage bowel outputs, a commonly home-based technique that offers the person with stoma between 12 to 24 hours of intestinal emptiness. Instead, my research participants must resort to the continuous use of ostomy bags, which sometimes fill up in a matter of minutes. Ostomy bags delivered by the NHS to my informants are beige, approaching 30 centimetres in length when rolled out and 5 centimetres wide for an adult size. They hold a maximum of 400–500 millimetres of faecal waste before overflowing. Plastic, flexible, and waterproof; the pouch is attached to the skin around the stoma with a flange. Of red-like colour, without innervation, and of variable diameter but usually round, the stoma is the measure against which the inner circle of the pouch flange must be frequently sized by the person to prevent the strangulation of the stoma. The flexibility of the flange not only offers support to the wall but also affords a tight fitting on the belly irrespective of the shape of the abdomen. Such flexibility is essential as people like Elizabeth develop hernias around the stoma, changing, in turn, the topography of the abdomen. Adhesive remover, wipes and skin protectors are used to avoid dermatitis or excoriation on the site in which the flange is glued. In cases of high-output colostomies, such as while the person is on chemotherapy, drainable stoma bags come in handy because watery waste is emptied without the need to detach the bag from the body. Users simply open the lock and roll closure mechanism at the bottom of the pouch.

Internally, the ostomy bag is coated with an odour-barrier film and contains a charcoal filter to deodorise and allow the escape of gas. However, filters sometimes become blocked with moisture from the faecal output, leading the ostomy bag to '*balloon*' and even blow-up. It is recommended that users pay attention to diet, practise slow and mindful chewing, and avoid raw vegetables and fizzy drinks that may cause bloating. Ruth, another research participant in her late thirties who was going through treatment for rectal cancer and had a permanent colostomy, knew exactly what foods had caused the stoma accident. On the chemotherapy suit and while having chemotherapy, she once ate a jacket potato with beans for lunch. We said goodbye, and on her way home after the infusion, her stoma ballooned, causing faecal leakage on the bus. The trade-off between adhering to a constipating diet and enjoying the food one eats is a constant tension that does not have a stable solution. Conversely, lack of air and constipation may cause *pancaking*, which accounts for a second cause of leakages. It happens when the consistency of stools is more solid, and matter sits at the entrance of the bag, collecting around the flange instead of sliding towards the bottom of the pouch. Unlike ballooning, pancaking is a common occurrence for people with stomas exhibiting a more stable bowel function, who are likely to be off chemotherapy. My research participants who were wearing ostomy pouches while on chemotherapy would always carry a case with few spares of each appliance in case they find they have to relieve themselves on the go.

Having described the main features of the surgical procedure and the material qualities inbuilt in ostomy bags, I will now focus on the ways in which it is possible to understand bowel control for people with stomas in their daily lives. In the following section, I will turn to a discussion of the practices that make up stoma care for the research participants in my study. Understanding stoma care through the material arrangements that afford patients bowel continence or mitigate the consequence of leakages during cancer treatment, rather than, say, psychological strength, provides an important point of contrast to discuss research findings on 'adjustment' explicitly advanced by clinical professionals. My argument is that psychological adjustment comes only after, not before, physical adjustment: A well-fitting stoma bag over healthy skin might, indeed, solve most of the problem, if conditions are provided. I will illustrate the socio-material conditions that allow people with stomas to achieve a sense of normalcy in their lives after bowel surgery by enacting a body synthesis of heterogeneous material elements.

Coping: coordinating a larger body

When I started fieldwork in 2015 in the gastrointestinal clinic, I was kindly received by two bowel cancer support groups in South England to discuss how they could help me improve the design of my study. As people who have learned to manage their stomas for years, they thought it was more useful for me to understand the ways in which they navigate the rhythms of daily life with a changed bowel function. Knowing what bowel cancer patienthood looked like in practice, they seemed to suggest, would help me improve the design of my research project. I took their piece of wisdom and transformed it in a decalogue.

- One's body will never be the same, and it is important to accept that, for even we ask why this happen to us, we must get on with life, for us and for the ones we care about.
- One plans for trips with stops in which a toilet in good conditions is hopefully available.

- One experiments with the design and the opening of the pouch until finding the right one.
- One learns to eat again; low fibre diets and little alcohol are the best to slow down peristalsis.
- One makes sure not to lift anything heavy and do only gentle exercise not to cause hernias and stoma prolapses.
- One finds the daily balance between having diarrhoea or constipation, depending on how much loperamide – thickening tablets – one takes.
- One washes the skin around the stoma with soap and warm water thoroughly to prevent excoriation.
- One reaches out to others in offline or online support groups, for their members will understand what one is going through.
- One reads '*Tidings*', the magazine for people with ostomies, to find more tips.
- One carries a change of clothes together with the stoma case, especially while on chemotherapy cycles.

The members of the support groups I attended were emphatic when explaining that the fear of 'accidents' seems to take one's life away, one's ability to go about with life, until one finds balance amidst the unpredictability of one's bowel movements. As the decalogue shows, balancing means tinkering with different material elements over time, such as food intake, their own bodies, public infrastructure, thickening tablets, bowel movement consistencies, clothes, and ostomy bags. By tinkering with the material forms of one's own body and its surroundings, one can gradually learn how to deal with an erratic and sometimes explosive bowel function during cancer treatments; this 'tinkering' will also slowly help the patient come to accept his or her body after surgery. Adjusting to the stoma is premised in the coordination of socio-material practices that can make bowel motility happen in a controlled way. Following Mol and Law (2004), I suggest that the way in which my research participants aim to continue with their lives despite and beyond cancer treatment depends on the enactment of a different and larger body, a body-with-stoma. The analysis must focus then on 'the body we *do*' in opposition to the 'body we *have*' or 'the body we *are*.' In other words, it is through the productive coordination of different material practices that one produces a body that is substantially different from both the anatomical body that is objectified by the medical gaze and our own representation of it as a component of our self-image. Undoubtedly, enacting 'the body we do' requires work, constituting an achievement when we are successful in keeping it coherent (Mol and Law 2004). Gaining 'coherence' enables one's bowel function and mitigates the inherent tensions embedded in managing one's life.

Managing the different materialities in the construction of the body with stoma requires time, and my research suggests that people are only able to 'accept' their body after such coordination is achieved. The process of tinkering or experimenting with materials precedes, then, the process of adjustment. Warnier (2001) advances a praxeological approach to understanding the relationship between the co-constitution of the subject and the material culture in which she or he is situated. Similar to Mol and Law's understanding of the 'body we do,' Warnier conceptualises the body as a heterogeneous material synthesis. In a more psychological enterprise, Warnier suggests that the subject incorporates experiences arising from its engagement with its material world through sensorimotor practices. Sensorimotricity, together with speech and images, are mediums through which the new (material) experiences of the world are internalised by the subject. This process of domesticating varying material experiences is what Warnier understands as 'symbolization' (2001:14), a process that enables the subject to find meaning in events that are unruly, or that misalign from the stereotypical ordinariness of the day-to-day. Temporality is an important feature implicit in this process of symbolisation that aims at normalising experiences that otherwise would have unexpected consequences. By means of reproducing, and at the same time reshaping, sensorimotor engagements, Warnier proposes that practice acquires meaning for the subject and that such practices are incorporated into a normal sequence of events. Stoma management is, for my participants, exactly this kind of repetitive and creative process of material tinkering that enlarges the body. Highlighting the materiality coordinated in this process bears important implications for our understanding of behaviour change in people who have gone through stoma formations. In the next section, I would like to argue what a material culture approach offers to our understanding of the ways in which people with stomas adjust to their anatomically transformed bodies.

The idealism of adjustment

People with stoma not only go through the struggle of maintaining a sense of the self while their bodies are unbounded, but also must learn and get acquainted to dynamics surrounding faecal incontinence while trying to go on with their lives. Both aspects are said to affect the emotional response that patients develop to the stoma post-surgery: the perceived lack of control or lack of acceptance triggering maladaptive practices that cause emotional distress (Ranchor et al. 2010). The degree of stress that living with diverted bowels generates in the person is what clinical psychologists understand as 'adjustment to stoma formation' (Simmons et al. 2007). Operationalised as a concept concerned primarily with the measurement of 'quality of life' for people with stomas, adjustment uses standardised metrics to understand the psycho-social burden imposed by the stoma formation. Patients' responses are rated on a scale that has become essential to understand both patients' needs and how they are supported by clinical professionals. The key explanatory variable usually incorporated is 'coping,' which, in turn, depends on two stages of cognitive appraisal. The first stage is about the nature of the stress, and the second is about what the individual thinks they can do to address it. Proponents from health psychology suggest that 'self-efficacy' predicts health behaviours (Ashford et al. 2010). However, 'self-efficacy' is a difficult behavioural construct to modify. This type of behaviour change is affected not only by external sources of motivation (if they are even available for modification), but also enduring affective states and physiological conditions (Bandura 1977). Therefore, it is possible to say that cognitive models of adjustment to stoma formations assume that the individual's reaction to estranged body parts depends on the interpretations she or he makes on the basis of the information that is available, and the extent in which they believe they have the skills to produce the effects (on the body) that are desired. The appraisal process, shaped by one's self-belief, explains how the individual responds to the stoma and its consequences.

The clinical use of 'adjustment' is then predicated upon the transference of control from surgeons and nurse specialists to patients through the clear and compassionate provision of information so they can 'self-manage,' a concept that underpins the responsibility of the individual to take care of their own health, which currently gaining much currency in the NHS in the face of an increasing demand for healthcare services and high work pressure for clinical teams (Foster et al. 2018). The premise is that patients will feel confident enough to manage the consequences of cancer and its treatment if they acquire the relevant knowledge to cope with the disease. Practical knowledge will enable patients to change their behaviours as needed and to make sense of the body-with-stoma as the 'new normal' (McVey et al. 2001). From this perspective, Jay was able to adjust to the stoma formation, partly because his own belief in himself and in his capacity to learn the skills necessary to achieve bowel control, whereas Elizabeth found it more problematic, as she did not feel confident either about what her own body could do or about her future. Through this lens, the achievement of coordinating 'the body we do' through the habituation of embodied skills, draws from absorbing and interpreting information that can, in turn, inform practical skills and changes in behaviour. The challenge, then, is that struggling to manage the pragmatic aspects of the stoma reinforced in Elizabeth a feeling of being out of control. For the colleagues working on psycho-social understandings of cancer survivorship (Foster et al. 2016; Grimmett et al. 2017), the problem for Elizabeth was one of self-efficacy: she was finding difficulty in self-managing her stoma because she did not believe if and how she could do it.

While acknowledging the relevance of people's psychological states to understand how they cope with stoma formations, I would like to argue that adjustment, as defined here, requires a more complex analysis that takes people's struggles seriously. Enacting 'the body we do' demands that one considers both the self-managing agent but also the context in which she or he is situated. Against the ideal of a self-managed patient who is proactive and knowledgeable regardless of the resources available to him or her, my ethnography provides context in which materiality precedes the attitudes of my informants. Regardless of the psychological states of my informants, efforts to help them self-manage the side effects of their cancer treatments must include access to infrastructure and economic support. We must interrogate the material affordances of cancer survivorship, that is, the possibilities for action through which materials allow a successful process of bodily synthesis for the enactment of the body we do. Simon's story is illustrative in making this point.

After a bout of uncontrollable abdominal pain, Simon decided to go to A&E, already considering the possibility that something was seriously wrong in his body. The medical doctors quickly referred him to the cancer clinic in which professionals determined that his cancer had already spread to the liver at the moment of the diagnosis. As a result, local surgery was no longer advisable, and chemotherapy was his only viable option. After the second cycle of treatment to deal with a non-resectable advanced sigmoid cancer with liver metastasis, another bout of pain and projectile vomiting overwhelmed him. His bowel had perforated, and emergency surgery was necessary to keep him alive. The procedure resulted in the formation of a temporal colostomy, so like Jay and Elizabeth, he had to learn to live with that. However, unlike Jay and Elizabeth, he did not enjoy the same material conditions or social support. Threatened to be made homeless by members of his family with whom he lived and having lost his zero-hour contract job after the cancer diagnosis, he was left in a very difficult position. The flat in which he was living with his close family belonged to his deceased father, but it had become the main source of family conflict. The dispute over the father's inheritance reached the county court. Until the judge could make a decision on the case, his mother and sibling determined that Simon was not allowed to use the kitchen for cooking or the washing machine to do the laundry, and he was prevented from using the toilet from midnight to 7:00 a.m. His relatives did not care that Simon had to deal with a stoma and chemotherapy at the same time, challenging him to contain the faecal waste by other means. At 50 years old, Simon was living under a curfew, and as the flat was locked from inside by his mother at night, he feared that an ambulance would not reach him should he require emergency care. His relatives observed strict silence with him – his mother simply did not want him to feel as if the flat was his home. They felt that using the toilet, the kitchen, or the laundry would allow him to feel a sense of ownership of something that was in dispute.

Simon considered his stoma to be the 'worst part of the cancer.' It leaked non-stop. He lacked the ability to do his laundry, to change his stoma bag at night, or prepare more suitable food at home. Moreover, he was suffering from an intestinal prolapse occasioned by carrying his heavy backpack every day. Because he could not trust his relatives in his home, he often carried around his laptop, all his hospital letters, and his medical appliances. During an appointment with the stoma nurse to which both of us went, we found out that his stoma had indeed prolapsed due to the heavy weight of the backpack, and that he was strangulating it because he was not measuring the bags correctly. He was not registered with the GP because his social situation prevented him from having a proof of permanent address, so he found himself recycling the stoma bags that the hospital had given him more than six months ago. In turn, the petroleum-based cream he was using to heal the skin around the stoma provoked an allergic reaction and excoriation, so the bag was not able to stick properly. A year later, the material constraint continued to oppress him; he lost his case in court, and found himself in an even more precarious position. Unlike Jay and Elizabeth, who fortunately did not face serious economic constraints and enjoyed the support of their families, Simon was not always able to produce the larger body-with-stoma and secure its optimum management. Despite his proactivity, he lacked the access to basic infrastructure.

Discussion

This chapter has tried to unpack the socio-material practices that make up the body-with-stoma in order to complement academic perspectives that understand the challenge of faecal incontinence from the point of view of its effects on the individual's self-image and integration in social dynamics. Drawing on three main ethnographic cases from colorectal cancer patients undergoing treatment in a teaching hospital in London, a rendering of stoma management has been offered that highlights its material aspects, proposing an analysis that sheds light on the preconditions of bowel control for people with stomas in everyday use. Hence, this approach has been developed to contribute to clinical understandings of processes of adjustment that otherwise tend to idealise proactive attitudes to stoma management under the possible slogan: 'more and better information for a supportive process of behaviour change.' Such an approach, currently used by stoma nurses in the clinical team, transfers responsibility from the clinic to patients irrespective of the material and economic support they find available. Interested in patients' quality of life, clinical professionals aim to give compassionate and informative advice. However, I have argued that the tensions that arise in the enactment of a body with stoma must pay attention to the material surrounding that enables colorectal cancer patients to live their lives despite and beyond treatment. Instead of focusing on patients' perceptions of lack of control, or disregard for the recommendations they receive from clinical professionals, it may be the case that 'maladaptive' behaviours are not just a consequence of individual attitudes. My ethnography shows, then, that well-fitting stoma bags over healthy skin solve most of my research participants' struggle if basic infrastructure is provided.

Acknowledgements

I would like to thank the research participants who generously shared with me their experiences of living with cancer and CONICYT/Becas Chile 2014 (72150288) for the financial support throughout my PhD studies in the UK.

References

Ashford, S., J. Edmunds and D. P. French (2010). What is the best way to change self-efficacy to promote lifestyle and recreational physical activity? A systematic review with meta-analysis. *British Journal of Health Psychology* 15(2):265–288.

Bandura, A. (1977). Self-efficacy: Toward a unifying theory of behavioral change. *Psychological Review* 84(2):191.

Cromar, C. D. L. (1968). The evolution of colostomy. *Diseases of the Colon & Rectum* 11(4):256–280.

Douglas, M. (2003). *Purity and Danger: An Analysis of Concepts of Pollution and Taboo*. London: Routledge.

Foster, C., L. Calman, A. Richardson, H. Pimperton and R. Nash (2018). Improving the lives of people living with and beyond cancer: Generating the evidence needed to inform policy and practice. *Journal of Cancer Policy* 15(Part B):92–95.

Foster, C., J. Haviland, J. Winter, C. Grimmett, K.C. Seymour, L. Batehup . . . D. Fenlon et al. (2016). Pre-surgery depression and confidence to manage problems predict recovery trajectories of health and wellbeing in the first two years following colorectal cancer: Results from the CREW cohort study. *PloS One* 11(5), e0155434.

Grimmett, C., J. Haviland, J. Winter, L. Calman, A. Din, A. Richardson . . . C. Foster (2017). Colorectal cancer patient's self-efficacy for managing illness-related problems in the first 2 years after 16 diagnosis, results from the ColoREctal Well-being (CREW) study. *Journal of Cancer Survivorship* 11(5):634–642.

Jacobs, M., J. C. Verdeja and H. S. Goldstein (1991). Minimally invasive colon resection (laparoscopic colectomy). *Surgical Laparoscopy & Endoscopy* 1(3):144–150.

Kuhry, E., W. Schwenk, R. Gaupset, U. Romild and H. J. Bonjer (2008). Long-term results of laparoscopic colorectal cancer resection. *The Cochrane Library*.

Lawton, J. (1998). Contemporary hospice care: The sequestration of the unbounded body and 'dirty dying'. *Sociology of Health and Illness* 20(2):121–143.

Lea, R. (2001). The performance of control, control as performance (Doctoral dissertation, Brunel).

Lewis, L. (1999). History and evolution of stomas and appliances. *Stoma Care in the Community* 1–20.

Loudon, J. B. (1975). Stools, mansions and syndromes. *RAIN* (10), 1–5.

Manderson, L. (2005). Boundary breaches: The body, sex and sexuality after stoma surgery. *Social Science & Medicine* 61(2):405–415.

McVey, J., A. Madill and D. Fielding (2001). The relevance of lowered personal control for patients who have stoma surgery to treat cancer. *British Journal of Clinical Psychology* 40(4):337–360.

Mol, A. and J. Law (2004). Embodied action, enacted bodies: The example of hypoglycaemia. *Body & Society* 10(2–3):43–62.

NICE. (2011). Colorectal cancer: The diagnosis and management of colorectal cancer. National Institute for Health and Care Excellence. Accessed https://www.nice.org.uk/guidance/cg131/documents/colorectal-cancer-full-guideline2.

Ranchor, A. V., J. Wardle, A. Steptoe, I. Henselmans, J. Ormel and R. Sanderman (2010). The adaptive role of perceived control before and after cancer diagnosis: A prospective study. *Social Science & Medicine* 70(11):1825–1831.

Simmons, K. L., J. A. Smith, K.-A. Bobb and L. L. M. Liles (2007). Adjustment to colostomy: stoma acceptance, stoma care self-efficacy and interpersonal relationships. *Journal of Advanced Nursing* 60(6):627–635.

Tao, H., P. Songwathana, S. Isaramalai and Y. Zhang (2014). Personal awareness and behavioural choices on having a stoma: A qualitative meta-synthesis. *Journal of Clinical Nursing* 23(9–10):1186–1200.

Thorpe, G., M. McArthur and B. Richardson (2009). Bodily change following faecal stoma formation: Qualitative interpretive synthesis. *Journal of Advanced Nursing* 65(9):1778–1789.

Tilley, C. (2007). Materiality in materials. *Archaeological Dialogues* 14(1):16–20.

van der Geest, S. (2007). *Not Knowing about Defecation*. Oxford: Routledge.

Warnier, J.-P. (2001). A praxeological approach to subjectivation in a material world. *Journal of Material Culture* 6(1):5–24.

4 The life course of labia

Female genital cutting in Somaliland

Caroline Ackley

This chapter is about Somaliland women's experiences of female genital cutting (FGC). I use the phrase 'female genital cutting' as opposed to 'female genital circumcision' or 'female genital mutilation' (FGM) to address linguistic misalignment and its consequences, as well as to avoid underrepresenting Somali women through 'a single story' (Adichie 2009) where their life experiences are reduced simply to those of their genitalia. Although this chapter takes women's labia as the foci of its analysis, it ultimately aims to shed light on the complexity of women's lives and the myriad experiences of FGC over the life course.

Much has been written about female genital cutting, and this chapter intends to problematise many representations and moral evaluations by foregrounding women's descriptions of FGC over the life course. Some focus their writing on descriptions of the 'pain,' 'suffering,' and 'sorrow' of female circumcision (Abdalla 2006) framed within a larger discussion of sexual violence and rape inflicted during the civil war in the 1980s (Gardner and El-Bushra 2004), whereas others take a strong political stance as anti-FGM campaigners (e.g. Edna Adan, Ayaan Hirsi Ali, Nimco Ali, and Layla Hussein). Some write about the moral debates surrounding genital cutting (Shweder 2000), including (the lack of) ritual (Hernlund 2000) and socio-historical embeddedness and beliefs (Hicks 1996; Van Der Kwaak 1992), and others write from their own experiences (Ahmadu 2000, Ali 2007, Dirie 1998). Boddy (1982, 1989) provides symbolic and ethnographic contextualisation of FGC through insight into women's moral worlds, and most recently (2016) challenges 'outsider' moral condemnation of the practice by drawing parallels with labiaplasty (see Giussy et al. 2015). Beyond these perspectives, other writers foreground the misalignment between international definitions of FGM and individual women's experiences (Conroy 2006, Vestbøstad and Blystad 2014). Still others examine health implications, prevalence rates, and change in practice (Gruenbaum 2013; Obermeyer 1999; Shell-Duncan 2001; Shell-Duncan and Hernlund 2000), including diaspora experiences (Jinnah 2015; Johansen 2016).

Building on these approaches to thinking and writing about FGC, this chapter considers FGC to be not only a key life phase for Somali women, but also something which takes on new meaning and is experienced in different ways during different life phases; in other words, FGC is neither a singular occurrence nor a static experience in women's lives. By building on a concept of the body as an 'inside' and an 'outside' (Cook 2007; Gell 1993; Strathern 1979; Benson 1997), where 'social and moral categories are based on the control of bodily flows' (Masquelier 2005:12) this chapter analyses the boundary created when women's labia are cut and sewn, stretched, ripped, and stitched during different life phases. It considers the material boundary the labia create, the fluids and physical things that pass through it, and the values associated with women's labia. The chapter concludes by suggesting that the physical folding in and opening up of the labia mirror the societal folding in of multiple moralities and the potential opening up of new opportunities for women.

FGC, values, and language

FGM and female genital circumcision are moral phrases that I specifically wish to avoid. The Somaliland women (and many others) who undergo this practice, who perpetuate this practice, or who advocate against it are not categorically good or bad. The practice of cutting one's daughter or granddaughter is influenced by, at times, competing and ethically assessed contradictory values caught in a tension that some urban and formally educated women have expressed in public and private discussions, and that I, an outsider anthropologist, have struggled with in attempts to understand why and how FGC is perpetuated. Women consider and negotiate international, religious, health, and gendered values as related to their bodies and their daughter's and granddaughter's bodies.

For example, in Somaliland, the *qabiil*[1] (clan) system of government (established in 1993) is heavily influenced by the international community, including international non-governmental organisations (iNGOs). The Somaliland government, in conjunction with large funding bodies like the United Nations, erects billboards and holds workshops condemning 'FGM.' Similarly, the parallel, 'traditional'[2] clan-nominated upper house of the government called the *guurti* or council of elders, which is heavily influenced by prominent Somali religious sheikhs and elders, also openly condemns 'FGM.' The *guurti* stand alongside 'modern' 'institutions of liberal democracy' – including the president, judiciary, lower house, and multiparty

---

1 *Qabiil* is also variably translated as 'tribe,' 'race,' or 'nation.'
2 Following Asad (1986), Masquelier (2009) and Soares (2000), I take Islam to be a discursive tradition, where tradition is 'a set of discourses that instruct how a practice is best secured and provides justification for why it should be maintained, modified, or rejected' (Masquelier 2009:9). In other words, any study of Islam is about practitioners' conceptions of 'correct' practice, including, as this article examines, FGC. For an alternative suggestion about the 'traditional' nature of the *guurti*, see Balthasar (2012).

elections (Rader 2016). However, in negotiating both 'traditional' and 'modern' influences, there is a slippage in discourse (see also Vestbøstad and Blystad 2014) that prohibits these two parallel systems of government from speaking to each other about what they each term 'FGM.'

The government and iNGOs consider FGM[3] to be any cutting, pricking, or modification of the female genitalia, whereas the *guurti* and religious leaders consider FGM to be only 'Pharaonic.' Pharaonic cutting is widely used in the literature and employed by Somalis themselves. It is believed the custom dates to the time of the Pharaonic Egyptians; however, this is debatable (Boddy 1982). Many Somalis believe that Pharaonic is prescribed in the Quran[4] (al-Munajiid 2005). Another term used in reference to this procedure is 'infibulation,' or 'type 3 FGM.' According to my informants, Pharaonic involves the cutting and removal of the inner and outer labia. It sometimes involves the removal of the clitoris, sometimes just the clitoral hood. The remaining skin is then sutured from the pubis towards the perineum, leaving a small hole (described by many friends as the size of a grain of rice or demonstrated as equivalent to that of the pinkie fingernail) in the vulva to pass menstrual blood and urine.

In Somaliland, the procedure is categorised as either Pharaonic or Sunna. For some women and girls, Sunna involves just the cutting of the clitoral hood, for others it is a complete removal of the clitoris. In other cases, after the clitoris or clitoral hood is removed, they describe three to six stitches that are made from the pubis towards the perineum, and meant to cover the area cut. Some women reported being told they were given Sunna by their mothers and grandmothers only to later learn they actually had Pharaonic, thus indicating a fluidity in the terms as related to type of cutting and number of stitches.[5]

The *guurti* and religious elders consider Sunna, not Pharaonic, to be obligatory; however, they previously considered Pharaonic to be the obligatory form of cutting.[6] In fact, this change in obligatory type of cutting,

---

3 Female genital mutilation is generally understood by the international community to comprise all procedures involving partial or total removal of the external female genitalia or other injury to the female genital organs for non-medical reasons (WHO, UNICEF, UNFPA, 1997).

4 See hadith narrated by al-Bukhaari [5889] and Muslim [257], Muslim [349], Abu Dawood [5271], *Fath al-Baari*, 10/340; *Kishshaaf al-Qinaa'*, 1/80, *Mawaahib al-Jaleel*, 3/259, *al-Tamheed*, 21/60; *al-Mughni*, 1/63, *Fataawa al-Lajnah al-Daa'imah* (5/223); see fatwas issued by Shaykh Jaad al-Haqq 'Ali Jaad al-Haqq, Shaykh 'Atiyah Saqar, *Dar al-Ifta' al-Misriyyah* (6/1986).

5 There is not necessarily consistency in description of Pharaonic and Sunna cutting. In women's descriptions of their experiences of FGC, sometimes the number of stitches determines which type she has, and other times, it is the amount that has been cut.

6 Women's campaigners, including local and diaspora Somalis, argue that it is due to the success of their advocacy and a change in Somaliland knowledge and sentiment towards the practice. Religious leaders argue it is due to a newly informed reading of the Quran and the Hadith.

from Pharaonic to Sunna, is in the process of becoming legalised. In February 2018, the Somaliland Ministry of Religious Affairs issued a fatwa (religious edict) banning two types of 'FGM': 'It's forbidden to perform any circumcision that is contrary to the religion which involves cutting and sewing up, like the pharaoh circumcision' (The Strategic Initiative for Women in the Horn of Africa, 2018). The fatwa also states that women who perform 'FGM' will be 'punished' and 'victims will be compensated' (Bhalla 2018); however, amongst prominent anti-FGM campaigners, there are significantly different interpretations of the fatwa's meaning and impact.[7]

The fluidity of terminology concerning Pharaonic and Sunna and the variation in their descriptions, along with the linguistic misalignment in the understanding of FGM, results in a slippage of discourse that creates, at times, conflicted and competing moral messages on cutting. Women receive messages from the outward facing 'modern' and 'intelligent' international community about the damaging and 'backwards' (see Carson 2016 for an interview with prominent Somali anti-FGM campaigner, Edna Adan) practice of any type of cutting. At the same time, they receive messages from the inward facing 'traditional' Somali Islamic authorities (*guurti* and elders) about the importance of practicing Sunna. These parallel messages create an idealised opposition involving recognised forms of knowledge and reasoning: Islamic knowledge and Quranic reasoning stand in opposition to biomedical knowledge and human rights reasoning; however, both sources of knowledge and lines of reasoning can end in a type of human flourishing predicated on belief of 'correct' Islamic and ethical practice and result in outward measures of success including formative experiences (schooling and wage labour), marriage, and family.

Inside and outside

The cutting of the labia minora and labia majora, and the sewing of the remaining flesh is not only a physical barrier between a woman's insides and outsides. It is also symbolic of her personal opening and closure over the

---

7 The Strategic Initiative for Women in the Horn of Africa wrote on their website, 'the fatwa of the [R]eligious [A]ffairs [M]inistry is misleading as it is not banning FGM from an Islamic religious view. On the contrary, it is allowing and legitimising type one FGM from an Islamic angle, which is still the most commonly practised type of FGM.' Similarly, Guleid Ahmed Jama, chairperson of Human Rights Centre Somaliland, said 'The decision of the religious ministry has effectively legalised FGM by only condemning two types of FGM. It has given a sense of religious meaning to something that has nothing to do with religion' (Bowman 2018). In contrast, Edna Aden tweeted her support of the fatwa and the ongoing struggle to eradicate 'FGM' worldwide (Bhilla 2018). Ayaan Mahmoud, Somaliland's representative in the UK, also welcomed the fatwa as 'a message from the government to everyone in Somaliland that there is no religious or cultural basis for FGM' (Bhilla 2018). She continues that it is 'a step in the right direction' although she is 'not completely satisfied with the fatwa' (Bowman 2018).

life course as substances and objects pass through her as well as a societal folding in of moralities and opening up of different ideals and opportunities. The physical barrier created by a woman's scar tissue acts as a 'border zone' (Benson 2000; Mattingly 2010, 2014) through which she is contained and protected from the outside world, yet, as substances and objects pass in and out, her sense of self is potentially vulnerable and she undergoes many transformations. For example, on a woman's wedding night[8] she is penetrated, possibly for the first time, by her husband. Her labia are ripped and stretched, often causing great anxiety and pain. She is vulnerable, and she may become pregnant – indicating a shift in her sense of self and social standing from wife to mother. In many ways, her body carries competing values: desirability and modesty, fertile strength and sexual passivity, autonomy and control. Her interior reflects[9] her inner piety, an inner ethical self. Her exterior self 'shines'[10] outward through her 'body, mind and spirit.'[11]

In considering the substances and objects that pass in and out of a woman's vulva over the life course, FGC can be analysed as more than a static experience, an experience that is only lived once at the time of cutting. Instead, women experience the physicality of having been cut and sewn differently at different life phases. They also understand the practice itself differently at the age of cutting (around age six) than they do when they begin menstruating, having sex, or bearing children. At each phase, the inside and outside are physically experienced and understood through a dialectical relationship between the self and the world; she gets to know her physical body and self in relation to the world through which she interacts and lives, while at the same time the teachings of the religious elders, the knowledge passed down from her mother and grandmother, and the influence of iNGOs, social media, and family living abroad all shape the way she understands and modifies herself. In other words, over the life course, the relationship between the inside and outside reveals that women are aware they have an 'appearance' that allows justifiable inferences about their moral character (Sacks 1972:281, 333).

FGC at different life phases

> *Women die three times: first, when they are cut; second, when they have sex on their wedding night; and third, when they have a child.*
>
> – Fowsia

8 Urban women often get married between ages 18 to 30, although this varies with education and economic class.
9 Here, I use 'reflects' metaphorically in relation to a woman's outward shine. However, see Gell's (1998:191–192) idea of the 'graphic gesture,' such that this may be constitutive of, not merely representational of, the woman's piety.
10 *Shidan* (slang).
11 As one teacher at Hargeisa's *Qoys Kaab* Islamic family and marriages classes taught a group of 50 unmarried secondary school and university girls between ages 15 and 25.

The phases described ahead represent friends' and informants' experiences of FGC over the life course. This scheme reflects the experiences of urban women (specifically those of Hargeisa and Borama) of varying educational and economic statuses: from those unable to read and write to holders of master's degrees, from house girls to the women they work for. This scheme is neither achieved by everyone, nor desired by everyone. For example, not all women will purposefully press the clitoris of their baby daughter, and not all women will get infections that require medical attention. However, this scheme does represent a myriad of women's FGC experiences as related to different phases of the life course.[12]

Baby

When a baby is born, the process of gendering begins. Warsame (2002) notes that in traditional pastoralist families, the news of a mother giving birth to a boy was often welcomed with a celebration. In contrast, 'discrimination' against girls incited women to compose songs and poetry that reflected their emotions towards the 'glorification' of boys and the 'undervaluing' of girls. Some mothers composed songs 'regretting' the birth of a daughter, whereas other mothers sympathised with their newborn daughters and expressed the 'unjustified treatment of women in general' (ibid: 33) through poetry.

The process of gendering is reflected not only in poetry and song, but also in the physical manipulation of the bodies of baby girls. Many mothers begin the process of physically gendering a baby girl by pressing her clitoris to prevent it from growing.[13] In an excerpt from my field notes, I write about a conversation with three women past childbearing age: Basr, Casha, and Casha's sister:

> *They say that when a baby girl is born the mother will take her home and massage her legs, she (Casha) shows me by rubbing her own legs then she says that the mother will make the baby calm and comfortable and then press her clit, hard. She shows me by using her thumb to press on her leg. She is pressing really hard, rubbing her thumb into her leg. She says the mothers do this to the baby girl's clit so it doesn't grow and show between her legs.*

12 Key phases in many Somali women's lives according to an 'ideal' model: (1) *afaartan bax* celebration 40 days after the birth of a child, (2) FGC, (3) wearing hijab to school, (4) beginning household responsibilities, (5) finishing reading the Quran for the first time, (6) first menarche, (7) secondary school, (8) university, (9) marriage and first sexual intercourse, (10) childbirth, (11) motherhood, (12) menopause, and finally (13) death of husband. This model illuminates transformations women undergo physically, spiritually, developmentally, and within the unit of the family.

13 For more on practices that change the body and being of babies, see Katz (1989) on uvulectomy across Africa and Warnier (2007) on moisturising with oil in Cameroon.

A baby girl's genitals are open and vulnerable; vulnerable to growing too large.

> *I then say that I read an article where a woman likened the clit to a man's penis.*[14] *She wrote that people believe that a girl becomes a woman when her clit is cut, that way she no longer metaphorically resembles a man.*
>
> *The women immediately discount this interpretation, saying it is not true. Then the sisters argue a little, the sister says that maybe the clit can protrude and they ask me what I think, does the clit look like a penis if it is left untouched? Basr and I tell them that no, in no way does it resemble a penis. They say that nobody thinks this.*

The women reveal their fear that the clitoris may protrude past the labia and resemble a penis, but upon hearing from two uncut women (Basr and me) that it does not they rest assured in their initial belief about what an uncut clitoris looks like. Their discussion shows that baby girls are open and vulnerable in the process of changing the body; however, the sculpting of the body is not necessarily about changing it away from something (being male), but changing it towards a better, more ideal, form of itself; thus enhancing virtue through material body shaping.

Girlhood

Until around the age of six most babies and young children live in the world of women. They are cared for by their mother and other women and girls in the house. It is only around age six that boys and girls begin to be separated. Many girls are cut *(gud)*[15] between the ages of six and eight; however, the exact age depends on many factors; including the *Gu* rains,[16] the return of family from abroad, and the schedule of the traditional birth attendant (TBA) or midwife. These factors often coincide in a 'cutting season' in the summer when the diaspora coordinate the cutting of their daughters with their urban and rural family; thus coordinating a time of plenty for rural family, with summer holidays for urban and diaspora family, in turn, facilitating the TBA/midwife's schedule.

One friend, Fowsia, who is considered an old woman now, still remembers very clearly the day she was cut. She began by explaining that she grew up just outside Hargeisa before the war.[17] She described a life of rural isolation,

---

14 Van Der Kwaak, Anke. 1992. 'Female Circumcision and Gender Identity: A Questionable Alliance?' *Social Science & Medicine* 35, no. 6: 777–87.

15 Also, *gudan, gudaal, gudniin.* Lit. circumcise, circumcised, circumcision.

16 This tends to be in April/May and is primary cropping season for agropastoralists.

17 The war Fowsia is referencing is the civil war which grew out of the Siad Barre regime's rule during the 1980s. Fowsia is considered an old woman and does not know when exactly she was born, but she was possibly in her 60s at the time of this research.

which is typical of villages outside of Hargeisa even today. She says she was cut when she was a young girl, she does not know when exactly, but it is likely she was between six and eight years old. As she told me about that day, her body language and her voice changed, suggesting a deep concentration in recalling something so intimate and painful that was so long ago, and a detachment from the visible trauma she experienced.

Fowsia was cut by a woman who stopped at her family's hamlet as she travelled the countryside cutting girls. Fowsia spoke of lying on her back and being held by her arms and her legs while the woman cut her clitoris first, then her inner labia, and finally her outer labia, all with a pair of scissors. The parts of her that were cut would have either been buried or thrown away like is common today. She was then sewn with a long, sharp, thorn about the length of a pinkie finger and the width of a straw.

Fowsia was sewn from the 'top,' near the pubis, 'down,' towards her vaginal opening. The woman used a thread of plastic from a large grain sack. The woman left a small hole near the vagina, the size of a grain of rice, for Fowsia to urinate from and pass menstrual blood when she was older.

Other, younger women, also described traumatic experiences. A long-time friend, Hodan, explained to me over coffee one day that her grandmother tricked her by telling her she was getting Sunna and only later did she learn she had Pharaonic. Hodan even made a drawing to clarify her understanding of the difference between Sunna and Pharaonic, namely the number of stitches (three stitches over where the clitoris was cut for Sunna, and six stitches or more for Pharaonic leaving a small hole to pass urine). Many other women recalled their experiences, each of them changing in disposition and voice, turning inwards as they described the cutting and the pain. Many of them emphasising the small hole remaining, often described by holding up their pinkie finger and pointing to the fingernail.

Of the women I met during the 18-months of research that inform this chapter, nearly all had what they would describe as Pharaonic, and only few claimed they had Sunna. One father, a colleague at an NGO I worked for part-time, proudly described the day his daughters were cut. He emphasised that they walked to be cut and even walked home from being cut. This signalled that his daughters were given Sunna instead of Pharaonic; namely because when a girl is cut according to Pharaonic she is immobile, with legs bound together, until she heals enough not to rip open the stitches nearer to the vaginal opening.

After a girl is cut and she is relatively healed, her new status as clean and (religiously) pure (in contrast, one mother described uncut women to me as 'dirty, dirty, dirty!') becomes known in subtle ways. One such way, which Hodan illuminated and then eventually became obvious, is the (lack of) sound when passing urine and the amount of time it takes to pass urine. Hodan explained that one can tell how many stitches a girl has by the sound she makes when urinating. If she makes no sound that means her hole is small, so small that only a trickle can pass and it will take her a long time to urinate (and she is susceptible to kidney infections from holding her urine). If she makes a loud sound that means her hole is big. The sound and length of time it takes a girl to urinate, according to Hodan, shows whether she has been cut and with what kind of cut.

Puberty

The size of a girl's hole not only restricts or enables the flow of urine, but also the flow of menstrual blood and clots. Women have difficulty passing menstrual blood *(caado qab* or *dhiig)*,[18] some reported large clots that eventually had to be surgically removed,[19] and others described frequent infections from trapped menstrual blood and clots. I was told that menstruation is extremely painful and often witnessed my friends crying in bed for several days with pain.

In *Qoys Kaab* Islamic family and marriage classes, Dr Shukri, a Hargeisa-based OB/GYN, gave a lecture on women's health and what she considered to be key life transitions in women's bodies: menstruation, childbirth, and menopause. After her lecture, experiences of 'normal' were discussed in the question-and-answer session. Menstruation was the topic most of the students were interested in presumably because, as women pre-marriage, this was the life change they had most experience of, and it was easier to ask about what they knew than the future changes they have yet to experience. One young woman asked, 'How much pain [is OK when menstruating]?' Dr Shukri answered that 'a little pain is normal, [but] FGM causes more pain. [For example] if you have to stop your job, it's not normal, but for Somali girls it is normal because we have FGM.'[20] She continued, 'I have never seen a Somali woman with a labia minora, but we don't need to cut. If [women] know the benefit of having [labia minora] when married, they may not cut [their daughters]. Pharaonic FGM threatens elasticity of the vagina. Your vagina will be hidden, and the hymen won't let your menstruation to come out. Causes of stress, like exams, give lots of pain during menstruation.'

Dr Shukri's answer that some menstrual pain is normal, but that Somali girls with FGM have a bad type of pain indirectly suggests that Pharaonic is bad for women's health, and that this pain should not be tolerated. This bad pain can lead to problems with pregnancy and childbirth, important phases in a woman's life. Menstruation not only signals a young woman's fertility, potential desirability, sexuality, and femininity, but also begins her

---

18 Lit. blood.
19 There are many women, and indeed many stories about women, who repeatedly develop infections from trapped menstrual clots. Some women go to the doctor and are surgically opened to remove the clots. One woman I met could be opened only after travelling to Djibouti, where the doctor removed a ball of clots the size of a grapefruit.
20 Dr Shukri lectured that urinary tract infections are also common for young women due to their 'FGM.'

cultivation of pain as a virtue, and the development of her skill to differentiate between good and bad pain.

Early adulthood

The potential pain of a woman's first sexual intercourse creates anxiety for many women. One woman, Asma, delayed her wedding day numerous times over a six-month period because she was so afraid of being opened, ripped, and stretched by her husband on their wedding night. Her fiancé nearly called off the wedding because of her delays. Another woman, Hini, said that on her wedding night, her husband tried to enter her, and she pushed him off screaming in fear. It was only several nights later that they had penetrative sex. For Hini, the pain of her hymen breaking was terrifying enough to risk rejecting her husband.

The anxiety of women's potential pain in the breaking of the hymen or the ripping open of scar tissue extends to the women's celebration *sabiib*, usually seven days after the wedding. I attended Hini's *sabiib* with several of her other friends. We went to her 'honeymoon house'[21] for tea, snacks, and sweets. Sometimes there is music and dancing, and there is always a *xeedho* – a hard basket *(sati)* with lid covered by a white cloth *(salaq)* and wrapped in twine or rope. Inside is often *muqmad* (small dried bits of meat) preserved in *subag* or ghee, with a thick coating of dates with spices and sometimes various wrapped sweets. It is meant to symbolise the high-energy and high-fat food a young nomadic couple would eat for the first months of their marriage as they moved through the countryside. The basket is skilfully wrapped by the bride's mother in twine and into a complicated pattern that is difficult to untangle; often, there is only one opening of the twine on the *xeedho*. The young groom must attempt to unwrap the twine in front of the young bride, her friends, and her female family. Any time he makes an error the bride's mother and female family will hit his hands with a stick, bringing him shame. The successful unwrapping of the basket symbolises his success at opening his wife on the wedding night. He is rewarded with sweet delicacies inside the basket, much like the pleasure had on the wedding night.

The playful nature of opening the *xeedho* does not reflect the seriousness[22] of opening a woman's vulva on the wedding night.[23] For women who

21 Upper-middle class couples, like Hini and her husband, will sometimes rent a house for several weeks or months after the wedding. It is hoped that the couple will conceive of a child during this honeymoon *(bisha malabka)* period.
22 One friend rightly chastised me for neither fully understanding nor capturing the fear young women have about the wedding night, 'this [being opened] is actually every girl's nightmare . . . this is [a] really sensitive and serious part of [a] girl's life and it definitely should not be taken lightly' (personal correspondence with Fadumo E., 9 February 2018).
23 Some women engage in sexual intercourse before the wedding night, others might have anal sex prior to getting married to preserve their FGC, and others will have oral sex. I also met a woman who had hymen reconstructive surgery and her FGC sewn tighter prior to the wedding night so her husband would not suspect previous sexual encounters.

have Pharaonic, the potential for pain can be terrifying. Numerous friends explained the various ways a woman can be opened, including penetration where the husband forces his penis, by the groom's mother (related to me as 'our horror story'), [24] or a midwife using a razorblade on the wedding night to make enough room for a penis to enter.

Sexual intercourse on the wedding night is very important for women. Hini explained that women in her family and the community expected her to be pregnant within three months of the wedding night.[25] Several women expressed a fear that if they do not get pregnant quickly that their husband will leave them or take a second wife. The pain of the first sexual intercourse is a pain that is virtuous and must be endured. Women transition from daughters to wives, and to potential mothers; each are key life phases that improve their social standing in the family.

Motherhood

The transition to motherhood is very important for women. A woman begins at the 'lowest' level when she first enters into marriage and her household duties are vast. As a woman has children, she will 'increase' in her household standing; her children will begin to take on duties, and if she lives with her husband's family, his brothers may take new wives who start at the 'bottom' and work their way up. When her children marry, the woman and her husband may live with the eldest son's family, where she will be relieved of many household duties and will have the 'highest' standing. However, to reach this important phase, a woman must first become pregnant and birth a healthy child.

The experiences of a friend named Idil summarise the difficulties many women go through to become mothers. Idil is the eldest of eight children and never went to school, so she grew up learning home-keeping skills and caring for her younger siblings. She met her husband, Ibraahin, in her neighbourhood. They decided to marry when they were in their late teens, what she herself described as 'young.'

Shortly after getting married, Idil became pregnant but had a miscarriage in the first trimester. She got pregnant again soon after the miscarriage, and again lost the foetus. Several months later she became pregnant and carried the baby to full term. Sadly, Idil experienced an obstructed and prolonged labour leading to an emergency caesarean, which resulted in a stillbirth.

She had had another miscarriage in the months following the stillbirth and eventually became pregnant again. We went to several pharmacies and doctors' appointments to make sure she would have a successful delivery. She suffered severe nausea and had medicines for multiple ailments I was not familiar with. With a group of friends, we managed to arrange a free

---

24 Personal correspondence with Fadumo E., 9 February 2018.
25 Hini became pregnant one month after her wedding night and now has a baby girl.

caesarean for her at the only public hospital in the country. Idil was able to successfully deliver her baby, a girl named Nadifa, who is doing well.

Idil, like many women I met, suffered difficulties trying to get pregnant. Then during delivery prolonged and obstructed labour were common problems according to many of the midwives I met in urban and rural areas. One midwife outside of Borama explained that many deliveries are obstructed due to undeveloped pelvis size of especially young mothers, and many times mothers suffer miscarriages due to undiagnosed infections related to FGC.[26] She also explained that during labour, when the baby is crowning, the midwife will make two small horizontal cuts on either side of the FGC hole. She said this is the best time to cut because the mother is already in so much pain that she will not necessarily notice the cutting. After the delivery, the mother is sewn. She explained that a mother is cut during the first three deliveries, but after that, the skin around her opening has become elastic enough that it is not necessary.

Fowsia's experiences mirror the description of the midwife. She began by recalling that she was on her back and being held down, much like when she was cut. A midwife held her arms while another woman tried to cut her scar tissue open with scissors. She said they cut when the baby is crowning and it is time to push it out. Fowsia kicked the woman with the scissors and refused to open her legs. She says more women came and held her legs so they could cut her open with small horizontal cuts on either side of her hole. The midwife then sat on her chest and pushed her stomach down, pushing the baby down and hopefully out. After the baby was born, they sewed her back up, like she was before.[27]

Menopause

The final phase in the life course of labia is menopause. During this phase, women are no longer fertile or sexually desirable, and it is understood as less of a physical transformation and more of a transition away from motherhood that alters women's relationships with their husbands. After menopause, women will reach a point in the life course where motherhood is no longer possible, and they will no longer endure menstrual pains or pains from intercourse and childbirth. Intercourse may no longer be sought because there is no possibility of childbearing, and this may prompt some men to seek a new wife. It is also a time where familial power relations transition, when women no longer need to fulfil the duties of bearing and raising children, and instead act as a potential mother-in-law who manages her daughter-in-law.

26 Obermeyer 1999 reviews the literature on female genital surgeries and calls for further research on the harmful effects of the practice.
27 For a comparison with the social construction of episiotomy in the UK, see Way (1998).

Although menopause was rarely, if ever, mentioned during conversation (only one friend expressed concern she might be approaching menopause), it was taught in *Qoys Kaab* Islamic family and marriage classes as an important physical transformation in the life course. Dr Shukri erroneously explained that after menopause, women would have less pain because intercourse and childbirth will open the circumcision and allow urine and old menstrual clots to pass.

It is also during this final opening of a woman's body that she can address the long-term infections that have plagued her. For example, Basr encouraged Casha to visit a doctor due to the recurring infection and fever she had experienced for several years. Casha had a cyst on her vulva the size of a golf ball opened and drained and was given antibiotics. Her status in the life course allowed her to overcome any shame in being opened.

A folding in, an opening up

> *Dhallinyaro waa rajo-ku-nool, waayeelna waayo-waayo.*
> *Youth live on hope, the elderly on nostalgia.*
> — Somali proverb (Bulhan 93, 2013)

The physical folding in and opening up of the labia over the life course takes many forms depending on the substances and objects passing through a woman's vulva as well as a woman's phase in the life course. The labia are opened, closed, stretched, sealed, and punctured. Urine, blood, and babies come out. Penises, semen, and sometimes medical tools like scalpels and scissors open and go in. A woman's labia becomes a border zone through which liquids and objects pass, and values become assigned reflecting the vulnerability of working towards an ethical self.

In addition to the bodily experiences of FGC, women experience a folding in of moralities and an opening up of different ideals and experiences. Through their bodies, they negotiate and balance competing moralities from the international community, friends and family abroad, religious elders, the *guurti*, social media, and television. The body, and FGC in particular, represents a folding in of moral discourses related to health, gender, and religion. These discourses are influenced by and learned through the passing down of intergenerational knowledge, iNGO activist agendas, friends and family living abroad and in Somaliland, social media and television, and by the constraints of poverty or the abundance of excess.

At the same time, women undergo a specific type of opening up to different ideals and experiences. When a young girl is cut, she may understand the reason as related to notions of piety, purity, and cleanliness, but when she is older, she may resent her mother or grandmother on grounds of health (mental and physical). For urban women, there is now the option for a doctor to cut open the scar tissue and issue a certificate of opening only if a male relative is present (although I never met a woman who did this because they feared their husband would not believe them). Through this new option women can forgo the potential pain of being ripped open by their husbands during intercourse. And many young men now desire a pleasurable sexual relationship with their future wives. They want their wives to enjoy intercourse, and for many men, they believe a girl with Sunna is much more likely to do so. These acts suggest that opening up is not just that of the bodily scar tissue but is part of a process composed of many social and moral layers.

Young women begin to think that something new may be possible, where action, and including others in action – husbands, mothers-in-law, doctors – facilitates a horizon of new opportunity to shape and imagine something different. However, such possibility shows how the processes through which women's bodies simultaneously transgress and reproduce a variety of socially enforced boundaries; namely, in the case of FGC, that many of the reasons women undergo FGC in the first place are related to the same reasons they must be accompanied by a male relative when opened by a doctor. Although this may not sit well with many, it is the uncomfortable reminder that women's bodily surfaces were, and still are, 'a central terrain on which battles for the salvation of souls and the fashioning of persons' are waged (Masquelier 2005:2).

The folding in of moralities, and the opening up of new opportunities, reinforces notions that gender remains a central axis of difference through which ideas of dirt, immodesty, and pollution have not only been historically instantiated (Douglas 1991), but also are fertile ground for challenging moral and social worlds (Masquelier 2005). Women's bodily surfaces can signify inclusion in society, whereas deviation from the (once) norm can lead to moral debate, deliberation, and negotiation with implications not just for an anthropology of the body but for wider political embodiment of medical materialities.

References

Abdalla, Raqiya D. (2006). My Grandmother Called It the Three Feminine Sorrows: The Struggle of Women Against Female Circumcision in Somalia. In Rogaia Mustafa Abusharaf (Ed.), *Female Circumcision: Multicultural Perspectives*. Philadelphia: University of Pennsylvania Press, 187–206.

Adan, Edna, Amal Ali, Abdirahman Mohamed, Thomas Kraemer and Sarah Winfield (2016). *Female Genital Mutilation Survey in Somaliland*. Report. Edna Adan University Hospital. Accessed 24 January 2018. orchidproject.org.

Adichie, Chimamanda Ngozi (2009). The danger of a single story. *TedTalk* 18:49. Accessed 15 June 2017. www.ted.com/talks/chimamanda_adichie_the_danger_of_a_single_story.

Ahmadu, Fuambai (2000). Rites and Wrongs: An Insider/outsider Reflects on Power and Excision. In Bettina Shell-Duncan and Ylva Hernlund (Eds.), *Female "circumcision" in Africa: Culture, Controversy, and Change*. Boulder: Lynne Rienner Publishers, 283–313.

Ali, Ayaan Hirsi (2007). *Infidel*. London: Free.

al-Munajiid, Shaykh Muhammad Saalih (2005). Circumcision of girls and some doctors' criticism thereof. Accessed 3 June 2017. https://islamqa.info/en/60314.

Asad, Talal (1986). *The Idea of an Anthropology of Islam*. Occasional Papers Series. Washington, DC: Center for Contemporary Arab Studies, Georgetown University.

Balthasar, Dominik (2012). State-making in Somalia and Somaliland: Understanding war, nationalism and state trajectories as processes of institutional and socio-cognitive standardization, unpublished PhD thesis, London School of Economics and Political Science.

Benson, Susan (1997). The body, health and eating disorders. In Kathryn Woodward (Ed.), *Identity and difference*. London: SAGE in association with the Open University, 121–182.

Benson, Susan (2000). Inscriptions of the Self: Reflections on Tattooing and Piercing in Contemporary Euro-America. In Jane Caplan (Ed.), *Written on the Body: The Tattoo in European and American History*. London: Reaktion, 234–254.

Bhalla, Nita (2018). Somaliland issues fatwa banning female genital mutilation. *Reuters* 07 February 2018. Accessed 07 March 2018. www.reuters.com/article/us-somalia-fgm-fatwa/somaliland-issues-fatwa-banning-female-genital-mutilation-id USKBN1FR2RA.

Boddy, Janice (1982). Womb as oasis: The symbolic context of Pharoanic circumcision in rural Northern Sudan. *American Ethnologist* 9(4):682–698. DOI: 10.1525/ae.1982.9.4.02a00040.

Boddy, Janice (1989). *Wombs and Alien Spirits: Women, Men, and the Zār Cult in Northern Sudan*. Madison, WI: University of Wisconsin Press.

Boddy, Janice (2016). The normal and the aberrant in female genital cutting: Shifting paradigms. *HAU Journal of Ethnographic Theory* 6(2).

Bowman, Verity (2018). Somaliland set to ban FGM but activists fear new law will fall short. *The Guardian*. 23 February 2018. Accessed 07 March 2018. www.theguardian.com/global-development/2018/feb/23/somaliland-ban-female-genital-mutilation-activists-fear-law-will-fall-short.

Bulhan, Hussein (2013). *Losing the Art of Survival and Dignity*. Bethesda, MD: Tayosan International Publishing.

Carson, Mary (2016). Edna Adan: 'With my army of midwives, fewer girls will go through FGM'. *The Guardian*. 12 December 2016. Accessed 14 May 2017. www.theguardian.com/society/2016/dec/12/edna-adan-with-my-army-of-midwives-fewer-girls-will-go-through-fgm.

Cook, Joanna (2007). Tattoos, corporeality and the self: Dissolving borders in a Thai monastery. *Cambridge Anthropology* 27(2):20–35.

Conroy, R. M. (2006). Female genital mutilation: Whose problem, whose solution? *British Medical Journal* 333(7559):106–107.

Dirie, Waris (1998). *Desert Flower: The Extraordinary Journey of a Desert Nomad*. Edited by Cathleen Miller. New York: William Morrow.

Douglas, Mary. (1991 [1966]). *Purity and Danger: An Analysis of the Concepts of Pollution and Taboo*. London: Routledge.

Gardner, Judith and Judy El-Bushra (2004). *Somalia – The Untold Story: The War through the Eyes of Somali Women, War through the Eyes of Somali Women*. London: Pluto Press.

Gell, Alfred (1993). *Wrapping in Images: Tattooing in Polynesia*. Oxford: Clarendon Press.

Gell, Alfred (1998). *Art and Agency: An Anthropological Theory.* Oxford: Clarendon Press.

Giussy, Barbara, Federica Facchin, Michele Meschia and Paolo Vercellini (2015). 'The first cut is the deepest': A psychological, sexological and gynecological perspective on female genital cosmetic surgery. *Acta Obstetricia et Gynecologica Scandinavica* 94(9):915–920. DOI: 10.1111/aogs.12660.

Gruenbaum, Ellen (2013). Female genital mutilation/cutting: A statistical overview and exploration of the dynamics of change. *UNICEF.* Accessed 30 August 17. www.unicef.org/media/files/UNICEF_FGM_report_July_2013_Hi_res.pdf.

Hernlund, Ylva (2000). Cutting without Ritual and Ritual without Cutting: Female 'circumcision' and the Re-ritualization of Initiation in the Gambia. In Bettina Shell-Duncan, Ylva Hernlund and Bettina Shell Duncan (Eds.), *Female 'circumcision' in Africa: Culture, Controversy, and Change.* Boulder, CO: Lynne Rienner Publishers, 235–252.

Hicks, Esther K. (1996). *Infibulation: Female Mutilation in Islamic Northeastern Africa.* New Brunswick, NJ: Transaction Publishers.

Jinnah, Zaheera and Lucy Lowe (2015). Circumcising circumcision: Renegotiating beliefs and practices among Somali women in Johannesburg and Nairobi. *Medical Anthropology* 34(4):371–388. DOI: 10.1080/01459740.2015.1045140.

Johansen, Ragnhild Elise B. (2016). Undoing female genital cutting: Perceptions and experiences of infibulation, defibulation and virginity among Somali and Sudanese migrants in Norway. *Culture, Health & Sexuality* 19(4):528–542. DOI:10.1080/13691058.2016.1239838.

Katz, S.S., (1989). Uvulectomy: A common ethnosurgical procedure in Africa. *Medical Anthropology Quarterly* 3(1):62–69.

Masquelier, Adeline (2005). *Dirt, Undress, and Difference: Critical Perspectives on the Body's Surface.* Bloomington: Indiana University Press.

Masquelier, Adeline (2009). *Women and Islamic Revival in a West African Town.* UPCC Book Collections on Project MUSE. Bloomington: Indiana University Press.

Mattingly, Cheryl (2010). *The Paradox of Hope: Journeys through a Clinical Borderland.* Berkeley: University of California Press.

Mattingly, Cheryl (2014). *Moral Laboratories: Family Peril and the Struggle for a Good Life.* Oakland: University of California Press.

Obermeyer, Carla Makhlouf (1999). Female genital surgeries: The known, the unknown, and the unknowable. *Medical Anthropology Quarterly* 13(1):79–106. DOI:10.1525/maq.1999.13.1.79.

Rader, Anna (2016). Verification and legibility in Somaliland's identity architecture. PhD Thesis, School of Oriental and African Studies.

Sacks, Harvey (1972). Notes on Police Assessment of Observable Character. In David Sudnow (Ed.), *Studies in Social Interaction.* London: Collier-Macmillan.

Shell-Duncan, Bettina (2001). The medicalization of female: Harm reduction or promotion of a dangerous practice? *Social Science & Medicine* 52(7):1013–1028. DOI: 10.1016/S0277-9536(00)00208-2.

Shell-Duncan, Bettina and Ylva Hernlund (2000). *Female Circumcision in Africa: Culture, Controversy, and Change.* Boulder, CO: Lynne Rienner Publishers.

Shweder, Richard A. (2000). What about female genital mutilation? And why understanding culture matters in the first place. *Daedalus* 129(4):209–232.

Soares, Benjamin (2000). Notes on the anthropological study of Islam and Muslim societies in Africa. *Culture and Religion* 1(2):277–285.

Strathern, Marilyn (1979). The self in self-decoration. *Oceania* 49(4):241–257.

Van Der Kwaak, Anke (1992). Female circumcision and gender identity: A questionable alliance? *Social Science & Medicine* 35(6):777–787. DOI: 10.1016/0277-9536(92)90077-4.

Vestbøstad, Elin and Astrid Blystad (2014). Reflections on female circumcision discourse in Hargeysa, Somaliland: Purified or mutilated? *African Journal of Reproductive Health* 18(2):22–35.

Warnier, Jean-Pierre (2007). The Skin-Citizens. In *The Pot-king: The Body and Technologies of Power*. African Social Studies Series. Leiden: Brill, 63–106.

Warsame, Amina Mohamoud (2002). *Queens Without Crowns: Somaliland's Women's Changing Roles and Peace Building*. Nairobi, Kenya: Life & Peace Institute.

Way, Susan (1998). Social construction of episiotomy. *Journal of Clinical Nursing* 7(2):113–117.

5   On 'being the problem'

The ontological choreography of the infertile male

Rebecca Williams

This chapter looks at what it is to be an 'infertile male' undergoing reproductive health treatment in the UK via a material analysis of its categorisation. Anthropology has a long history of looking at systems of classification to provide insight into how people construct their social worlds and the things within them. Traditionally, systems of classification and types of categories were studied in order to prove and understand variations in cognition (see Morgan 1871) and social structure (see Lévi-Strauss 1958). More recently, attention has been paid to how categories are defined in order to explore how people construct knowledge, and how these constructions shape experience (see Latour 1987, 1993[1991]; Strathern 1992; Martin 1991; Butler 1990, 1993). This ethnography contributes to this ongoing body of work by providing insight into the construction and position of the category of 'male' in line with a clinical diagnosis of infertility in a UK-based reproductive health unit (RHU).

The development of assisted reproductive technology (ART) created new opportunities for the study and theorisation of systems of classification. Within this arena, kinship, an area of study traditionally carried out in small, pre-industrial communities, was suddenly unfolding in a 'new' way under 'new' conditions (Strathern 1992; Carsten 2001; Franklin and McKinnon 2001; Franklin 2006). Euro-American kinship systems, that which constitutes 'family' life, were deemed the product of an established conceptual parallel of biological and social life – which ARTs challenged with the development of new 'hybrid' kinds, such as 'artificial life' (Strathern 1992:3–4). New ARTs were predicted, therefore, to produce not only 'new' ways of being in relation but also 'new' ways of *being*. The issue of *being* an infertile male undergoing fertility treatment has been previously addressed by a number of researchers over a variety of contexts (Dyer et al. 2004; Inhorn 2004, 2012; Goldberg 2009; Parrot 2014). Much of this research suggests, however, that the foretold collapse of traditional systems of classification and proliferation of 'new' ways of being, alongside the uptake of new reproductive technologies, has not come about (Becker 2000; Thompson 2005; Inhorn 2012). Instead, local categories such as biology and technology, nature and culture, male and female, sex and gender, are carefully maintained to uphold intersubjectively recognisable ways of being. This ethnography forefronts the material processes employed in the RHU to demonstrate the strategies involved in upholding the carefully constructed position of the infertile male.

To describe this, I will employ the term 'ontological choreography,' which Thompson (2005) uses to refer to the dynamic coordination of things, typically conceptualised as of different 'kinds,' in a way that preserves their ontological integrity. Ontological choreography goes on to some extent in all spheres of human activity but is particularly striking in ART implementation as it is a practice which confronts and challenges the boundaries of assumed natural categories. In addressing the construction of the category of 'infertile male' in this context, my use of the term 'ontology' will take a slight divergence from the Heideggerian stance, collapsing the traditionally ontological – the reality of being – with the epistemological – the construction of reality. The application of ontology in this way is an attempt to avoid devaluing experienced reality when discussing its construction, which is a risk when discussions are considered to hinge on the distinction between described ontologies and a tacit meta-ontology of its own (Pedersen 2012). Through the careful analysis of clinical practice, and reflective accounts collected in interviews,[1] the ontological choreography of nature and culture, sex and gender, self and relational other, through which the category of 'infertile male' is constructed, will be revealed.

Doing 'their bit'

In comparison to female reproduction, male reproduction is a significantly understudied area of research (Culley et al. 2013). The omission of male experience from fertility treatment research is a reflection of the industry in which it is conducted (Hudson and Culley 2013). Policy, funding, and institutional operations repeatedly mask the male role in reproduction. The RHU where this ethnography takes place proved no exception to this with most men attending as an 'addition' to their partner's fertility. This sidelined role was made manifest in clinic documentation, spatialisation, and procedure, which will be mapped out in the next few paragraphs.

The RHU where this study was conducted was one of only a few in the UK offering Andrology (specialist male health) services. Despite this, the majority of male diagnostics conducted in the Andrology laboratory were at the request of the Gynaecology Department or the IVF Unit, not at the behest of male health services. This was always, at least in the cases I observed, at

1 Data was collected over a ten-month period, working five hours a week in the male-focused branch of an undisclosed RHU in the UK. This primarily consisted of observation of patient/ clinical interactions in the Outpatients unit and diagnostics laboratory, building case studies of couples undergoing treatment and mapping their journeys through services, and informal conversations and in-depth interviews with both staff and patients.

a late stage in female exploratory procedures when there had been no con-
clusive evidence for female factor infertility or, when female factor infertility
was determined, in preparation for IVF. The absence of the male half of the
couple undergoing fertility treatment, up until this point, was made apparent to me through the vast number of men, referred to Andrology, who
required registration as new patients despite the fact they had been attending
the RHU for a number of months, even years. Throughout the RHU, clinical
files were registered to the female, who clinicians addressed as the primary
patient, and any assisted reproductive techniques were usually operationalised in her body. On occasion, even clinical undertakings performed outside
of her body were conducted in her name, evidenced through the number
of Andrology referrals and even results letters in her name: 'Dear Mrs Lisa
Colth, the results of your semen analysis indicate. . . .' The autonomous
patient so essential to bioethical practice (Muller 1994) was incompatible in
an arena where the ultimate aim, conception, required the management of
two bodies simultaneously – so the female body was centralised while the
male body was sidelined.

The absence, or invisibility, of the male body in this context reflected
more than its corporeal role in reproduction. Regardless of the corporeal
differences between reproductive bodies, attending to the female body prior
to the male was medically unjustifiable. In the UK, male factors contribute
to 52% of infertile couples, and it was reasoned by Andrology staff that
conducting Andrology diagnostics as soon as either member of the couple
was first referred to the RHU would have saved time, money, and excessive
invasive investigation into the female body. In light of this, Hudson and Culley (2013) conclude that the sidelining of the man in ART implementation
is the result of not medical necessity but of the hyper-medicalisation of the
'problematic' female body.

The position of the female body in the RHU was the product of a long
history of systemic operations that imposed unequal gender categories onto
sexed bodies. Here, 'sexed bodies' refers to cultural mapping of the binary
categories of male and female onto bodies that perform particular differenti-
ated roles in reproduction. Gender is now widely recognised as something
multiple and fluid, but no matter how the individuals attending clinic identified, the binary of male and female was both required and reinforced by
RHU practices; ART, a process in which ultimate aim is conception, requires
the fusion of what are identified as male and female gametes in order to a
produce offspring – a zygote. This process meant that these sexed bodies
took on gendered inequality in their positions and management in clinic.

Determinants of body categorisation and positionality began to be
explored through comparative ethnography in the 1970s. One of the most
seminal of writings of this time was Ortner's (1974) *Is Female to Male as
Nature is to Culture?* In this, Ortner claimed that across societies, the systemic undervaluing of women was apparent, and that gender stratification
was based on a fundamental opposition between nature and culture. Ortner

proposed that women, as a result of their reproductive functions and their role in the creation of life, were intimately associated with nature, and were, therefore, in need of careful management; men, for their part, were associated with culture and the creation of society.

The universal application of Ortner's argument, as well as the claimed relations between female-nature and male-culture, have been challenged ethnographically; the spheres of nature, culture, public and private, and the homologies posited between these categories and gender difference proved to be historically and culturally variable. However, the structuralist assertions made regarding the binary categorisation of male to female and nature to culture hold true within the context of the RHU. The female body was problematised whilst the long-standing privileging of the male role led to the male body's elevation beyond the realms of medical management (Hudson and Culley 2013). It was the systemic positioning of identified male and female bodies that led the RHU to overlook male reproductive disruption in its focus upon the problematic female body. This was evident in clinic documentation and the referral and results processes.

The hyper-medicalisation of the female body and invisibility of the male body were reinforced through clinical practices dependent upon their differential bodily roles in reproduction. While male bodies remained detached from the majority of medical protocols in fertility treatment, their partners' bodies assumed the sole role of patient. Busy work-life schedules often meant women attended the RHU without their partners for routine appointments or as they underwent invasive procedures and hormone therapy. Men were not needed for these procedures, as their bodily role in ART was limited to the acquisition of the male gamete, and they quite often came into clinic only to do 'their bit.'

Despite the claims men made of the importance of 'doing their bit,' the 'ease of it' was often positioned alongside the extreme experiences of women having to undergo invasive medical treatments. As one couple recounted:

WOMAN: *Such a fuss over that one bit, you'd have thought he was going to give birth.*
MAN: *Well yeah, it was important.*
WOMAN: *Yeah, but if my eggs had been crap then it wouldn't have mattered, would it?*
MAN: *Yeah, but it's the same isn't it.*
I mean your egg my sperm.
WOMAN [speaking simultaneously]:
Yes, but I had injections and drugs and all sorts to get my eggs.
I mean I know we're both needed but come on,
You do that most days.

They both laughed, but this was an aspect of treatment that many men when interviewed often expressed as 'pressured' and 'stressful.' The production of an ejaculate for semen analysis brought the male body into sharp focus. The male body, that had until now remained hidden to the clinical gaze, was suddenly in the spotlight, but the sexual connotations of ejaculation associated with masturbation prevented the social identity of the man from falling completely into category of patient (Becker 2000; Thompson 2005). The 'routine act' of masturbation sexualised procreation in a way that was not 'true' of the female body, requiring the process of semen collection to be dislocated from male desire and realigned with the hyper-medicalised female body so that men effectively became 'ejaculatory extensions of their partners' (Thompson 2005:128).

The process by which male ejaculation became an 'extension' of the medicalised female body was one that was carefully staged through spatialised practices in the clinic. The clinic, as a defined and conceptualised place, is the product of the complex interactions between space, knowledge and power that led to shift in surveillance practices culminating in the seventeenth century (Foucault 1995[1975]:195–228). During this time, patient-directed care became subverted with the advancement of new epistemic cultures that were to become the core of developing clinical medicine. Redefined power relations that came with the development of medicine allowed for the accumulation of new formations of knowledge, the development of which relied on spaces of regulated investigation (Foucault 1995[1975]:226). The aesthetic of these specialised spaces was such that their environment could be recreated across various contexts, so that the production of knowledge might be repeated and therefore gain authority as substantiated fact (Knorr-Cetina 1999).

The RHU was one such space. Composed of smooth lines, sharp forms, pastel-block coloured walls, wipe down surfaces, and grey laminate floor, it promoted ideals of cleanliness and the containment of pollutants – a clinical aesthetic, the effects of which have been well documented (Katz 1981; Rawlings 1989; Mody 2001; Lynch 2017[1985]). Waiting areas, consultation rooms, and procedure rooms all followed this decor, ensuring the removal of the personal through the elimination of 'homeyness' and all the social relations that this creates (see McCracken 1989:178). This spatialisation promoted a breakdown of the usual boundaries of public and private in a designated medical space. Most consultation rooms were composed of a 'desk-space' and a 'procedure' area, separated only by a thin, blue disposable curtain, allowing for very intimate, bodily invasive activities to be carried out by almost complete strangers.

Almost all female body investigations and interventions were carried out in these spaces; behind the curtain, women would undress from the waist down and lie on their backs with their legs in stirrups. Here, diagnostics, egg retrieval, and implementation were all conducted at the behest of the medical practitioner. The corporality of their reproductive functions ensured their medicalisation, as they were encouraged to become passive objects in their reproductive activity. In contrast to this, men had to take an active bodily role in 'doing their bit' as the production of an ejaculatory sample required masturbation and the control of the male body by themselves, on their own.

When it came to 'doing their bit,' the sexualised male body, so far invisible to the medical gaze, did not fit in these specialised spaces of knowledge production and medical authority. Instead the RHU had two Production Rooms dedicated to the making and collection of an ejaculatory sample. Here, there was no curtain with a medical practitioner waiting behind it for you to get undressed, rather men were expected to attend to themselves in private. The Production Room was a contested space – partially a continuation of the hospital decor, but it included a 'homely' single wooden bed and a wooden bedside table full of erotic magazines. As such, it was caught somewhere between the sterility of medicine and the dirtiness of a teenage boy's bedroom. Whilst the magazines and the furniture reflected the sort of arena in which this type of activity might usually take place, the white walls and plastic floor, clinical bins and rubber covered mattress reminded occupants that it was a space of medical practice, corralling the act within the medical realm. Once finished, their sample was returned to the reception where it would then be sent off for diagnostics, frozen, or used in IVF.

Through practices of patient documentation and sample collection, the male ejaculate underwent a carefully staged detachment from the unmanageable male body to be realigned with the hyper-medicalised female body as part of her reproductive process. The positions of the male and female body were sustained, in part, by the systemic hierarchies through which they were constructed. What is apparent, however, is how clinical practice not only maintained these positions, but also reinforced them. Existing clinical ethnography highlights how medicalisation acts as a mechanism in the production of systematic categories, through the bodies, institutions, and societies where medicine is practised. Waitzkin's (1984) ethnographic study of clinician/patient interaction identified clinical space as an arena in which the dominant ideologies of society were reinforced; class, race, and gender inequalities played out in interactions and were strengthened through the authority of medical knowledge (Lupton 1997:96). In this vein, RHU practices regulated and normalised the sexed body as that which performed a specific role in reproduction: male bodies came to be defined by their ejaculatory function, by 'doing their bit.'

Being 'the problem'

The sidelining of the male reproductive role in the RHU is mirrored in its role in infertility research. Infertility is a contested concept. Cross-cultural and Western minority population research has demonstrated the fluidity and contextual nature of notions driving action directed to improving fertility outcomes. For example, work in pronatalist, patriarchal societies show how the inability to produce a son is experienced as a fertility failure, and in communities where children are expected to quickly follow a marriage, invasive

fertility treatments are sought almost immediately after beginning unprotected intercourse (Culley et al. 2013:228). Normative assumptions of the
burden of reproduction being a 'woman's issue' are endorsed in research by
the complete occlusion of male factor infertility from demographic method.
According to the WHO, infertility is defined as when a woman of reproductive age lacks the ability to become or remain pregnant (Zegers-Hochschild
et al. 2009). This means that work exploring the meaning of infertility are
almost exclusively based on female perspectives and little is known about
how men may constitute fertility across societies, or what its disruption may
mean for them as they position themselves socially. This next section outlines how infertility was perceived and constructed within the RHU.

The International Committee for Monitoring Assisted Reproductive
Technology (ICMART) and the World Health Organization (WHO) have
now set a global standard for biomedically defined infertility as a failing
to conceive after 12 months of regular, unprotected intercourse (Zegers-
Hochschild et al. 2009). This standard applies to both sexes, and yet none
of the men first attending clinic considered themselves infertile, despite the
majority having failed to conceive for more than 12 months. As most men
were attending as 'additions' to their partner's fertility, very few of them
even conceived of the fact that they might be 'the problem' when it came
to getting pregnant. In fact, many men gave their ejaculatory samples with
the expectation that IVF would be performed with the contents, only to
be told it was not possible from the sample. It was only upon receiving a
diagnosis that these men began to comprehend that they could be infertile;
it was only then that they, as one physician remarked, 'grasped the reality
of the situation.'

With diagnosis, men were offered the 'truth' of the situation in the form
of a particular knowledge about themselves. In studies of health knowledge, social scientists have long distinguished between the 'physical realities'
of disease and the 'social constructs' of illness in order to understand the
'reality of the situation' is experienced. This approach has been criticised,
however, as reducing knowledges to mental images, representation, and cultural productions. More recently, attention has been turned to how these
knowledges are *performed*. The term 'performance' entered social sciences
for describing the ways people staged identities, and it was later used to
demonstrate the way reality is staged (Mol 2008:82). Reality is experience
as constructed through various frames of reference. These frames are the
product of our accumulative knowledge about the world. This is not an
activity of the human mind but of the body, created through various objects
and their performance. Analysis of performance allows for an engagement
with the material culture of medicine in order to understand how disease is
constructed and, in turn, impacts the reality of illness (Mol 2008:84). The
following analysis of the carefully managed performance of the substance
of the male ejaculate reveals how a diagnosis of male infertility was constructed in clinic.

Diagnosis requires the isolation of abnormality. In the context of Andrology diagnostics, this meant the abnormal contents of the male ejaculate. Investigatory medicine fragments the body so that the 'reality of the situation' can be determined not as that which is experienced by the patient, but by isolated body parts and their functions. In the RHU, this process began prior to sample collection, as men were given careful instruction on how to prepare their bodies in order to produce the 'best' possible sample. This included avoiding alcohol, caffeine, and recreational and therapeutic drugs as well as abstaining from ejaculation at least two days prior to sample production. When giving the sample, they were asked not only to confirm that they had refrained from this list of activities but also to document how much of the total ejaculation was collected, and whether the sample included the beginning, middle, and end of the ejaculation. This process was explained by clinicians in that they were 'not looking for [the patient's] day-to-day ability to conceive, but their ultimate capacity to conceive' and that they needed to 'see them at their best.'

In order for the 'ultimate capacity to conceive' to be known, the object of study (the male ejaculate) needed to become disassociated from its social environment. The process through which a thing, or person, is removed from its relational situatedness, to reveal its unbiased form, is one of 'purification' (Latour 1993[1991]:13–48). Purification entails a complex cultural practice based upon the understanding that the world is product of empirical 'truths' to be uncovered. This practice was made possible in the context of the RHU as it performed within a world composed of the defined domains of nature and culture. Cosmologies that comprise distinct ontological orders such as nature and culture, allow for things – existing in these different orders as 'kinds' – to be known and mastered (Hacking 1995). By creating a controlled environment through which the male ejaculate came into being, it shifted from a 'human' to a 'natural kind': an entity possessing properties bound by natural law that could be objectively known.

As a 'natural kind' the male ejaculate needed to be handled in such a way as to preserve its integrity and ensure no human interference; this was achieved by managing its performance through and in spaces so excessively humanised that they 'failed to be human' (see Tilley 1997:34). Transparency, of action and artefacts, was considered a vital aspect in allowing for sample performance at each step of sample processing. Although semen production was completed in private, the sample was required to be in a see-through plastic pot. Once labelled with patient details, surname underlined, this was placed in a see-through plastic wallet. Samples would be kept in a visible place in clinic until collected by a member of laboratory staff. In the laboratory, whenever a sample is handled, opened, or transferred to different storage facility, the documentation must be countersigned by staff. All laboratory equipment in which the sample was housed was made of clear plastic or glass. The laboratory, as a social creation identified as a physical space in which particular knowledges are produced, carries systemic weight in the production of scientific fact; operating as an 'enhanced' environment that 'improves upon' natural orders (Knorr-Cetina 1999:26). As objects enter this space, they become installed in a carefully controlled field so that they may be dissected, categorised, and normalised. In the Andrology Laboratory, the male ejaculate was 'cleaned and filtered' – meaning the semen were killed to prevent movement and then diluted – before a minute amount was placed in the Hemacytometers. The Hemacytometer was, to my untrained eyes, a clear plastic slide that contained two tiny chambers. When viewed through 1000x magnification, these chambers were marked with a grid where the immobilised semen could be counted. Even at this magnification, counting was difficult, so images were taken and from these morphologies was determined. These images were then stored on the hospital database under the patient's name: a permanent record of the properties of their ejaculate.

The results of the laboratory investigation were then presented to the clinician in a typed document that included the presence and morphology of spermatozoa in sample, the concentration of the dilution of the sample, and the normal range of spermatozoa expected in a sample of that dilution. This knowledge was then presented to the patient by the clinician. In the Andrology Outpatients clinic, rather than presenting the results as they were printed, it was often expressed as a range or a likelihood: 'Your count came back as very low,' 'The chances of conceiving without intervention are really not very good,' and 'I won't say there isn't a chance, but we must recognise that it's very a low chance.' It was this diagnosis, as particular form of knowledge, that both explained the past, the years of non-conception, and the future in terms of a prognosis of zero to little chance of conceiving with or without technological intervention. It was in this manner that men came to the realisation that they were, in fact, 'the problem' when it came to conceiving.

Being 'the problem,' however, was not solely reliant on a diagnosis of a 'small' or 'very small chance of conceiving naturally.' The experienced reality of an infertility diagnosis was sustained only as long as it was partnered with biological childlessness, and for many men attending, this was only a temporary state: some men attending had already fathered biological children without ART intervention, and many men who had a 'small chance' of conceiving naturally went on to become biological fathers either through IVF or ICSI. Intra-cytoplasmic sperm injection, or ICSI, accounts for 52% of the cases of insemination performed in the UK (HFEA 2013). ICSI can be performed with a single sperm and, although samples are usually 'washed and spun at high speed to ensure only the most healthy and active sperm are selected,' the manual manipulation of ICSI means that the mobility and morphology of the sperm do not 'matter so much.' Because IVF and ICSI are performed so interchangeably, success rates are no longer separated (ibid) From this, we can assume that 32% of the men in clinic who received a diagnosis of infertility that did not include the complete absence of sperm went on to father biologically related children. Even men whose ejaculations had not yielded enough, or even any, sperm for ICSI to be undertaken were able to undergo extensive treatments in order to recover even the smallest number of spermatozoa via hormone therapy or Testicular Sperm Extraction (TESE) – the process of removing a small portion of tissue from the testicle under local anaesthesia and extracting the few viable sperm cells present. This meant that, for many men, being 'the problem' was a transitional phase to be managed, but as long as a diagnosis of infertility and childlessness co-existed, the reality of infertility was experienced.

When diagnosis and non-conception did not align, when men experienced childlessness without a diagnosis or when men received a diagnosis of infertility but conceived a child, the two forms of knowing infertility – experience and pathological diagnosis – were incompatible with each other. This incompatibility was not due to a mistranslation, but was a practical matter. Mol (2000) explored the practical matters of medical knowledges to demonstrate that incompatibilities are not unbridgeable but political. By the looking at knowledges of disease/illness as they were performed by laboratory clinicians and by patients and doctors, Mol identified how inconsistencies between the two were overcome when the 'reality of the situation' was defined through politically validated systems of knowledge. In Andrology, for the majority of men, their infertility was not real until confirmed by pathological diagnosis. Likewise, the pathology of infertility was validated only when accompanied by the experience of non-conception. Here, we see the blurring of the boundaries social science has traditionally drawn between disease and illness (Kleinman 1980) as the physical realities of biomedicine (disease) and the social dimensions of these realities (illness) are unable to perform outside of each other.

Through the carefully controlled performance of the male ejaculate, the 'truth' about the man's 'ultimate capacity to conceive,' or the 'reality of the situation,' could be known. But the reality of infertility neither existed prior to diagnosis, nor was it a sole result of diagnostic techniques; it was a performance of male relationality that had undergone a process of purification so that its 'true' capacity – that deemed to exist in the natural order of things, prior to social relations and their effects – might be known. The formation of the male ejaculate required its removal from its 'social' settings in order for it to be dissected, categorised, and normalised, enhancing the powers of the clinician as they became the primary holders of its knowledge (Knorr-Cetina 1999:29–32). Once separated from the body the ejaculate acted as an object through which its ultimate capacity could be understood. This knowledge was then relayed to the patient as their ability to produce that which was needed in order to partake in the natural process of procreation. It was, however, only when this knowledge was accompanied by biological childlessness that it became politically validated.

Being an infertile man

Analysis of the material processes of undergoing a diagnosis of male infertility have, so far, demonstrated how men attending clinic were reduced down to a marginalised role in reproduction, that of providing the male ejaculate, and how the male ejaculate was managed in order to produce knowledge of a man's capacity to conceive. Fausto-Sterling (1995:127–134) cites scientific texts that construct conceptions of what it is to be 'naturally male' as an example of 'how to build a man.' In the same respect, the practices of Andrology diagnostics could be seen to be an example of 'how to reduce a man to their ultimate relational capacity.' In this context, a man's relational capacity came to be defined by the act of providing semen, knowledge of which changed the 'reality of the situation.' This was apparent in the way, upon reflection, men divided their time and experiences into 'pre' and 'post' diagnosis. Activities like masturbation, sex, and 'being a good husband' changed from being something they 'just did' – as an inherent part of their male capacity, to something that felt 'pressured' and 'embarrassing,' that they 'struggled to perform.' These actions, once 'natural,' came to symbolise how 'useless and pathetic' they were.

The effects diagnosis had on male relational capacity is supported by research demonstrating that, as much as masculine identities are multiple and fluid, they appear intrinsically tied to paternal achievement (Inhorn 2004:168–169). The *Oxford English Dictionary* defines 'male' as 'of or denoting the sex that produces gametes, especially spermatozoa, with which a female may be fertilised or inseminated to produce offspring' (*OED* 2015). In 'doing their bit,' male bodily capacity to produce the male gamete, previously hidden from the medical gaze, was suddenly in question. In a context where conception was the ultimate goal, men were confronted with their own 'maleness' in a way that might not be reflective of their everyday experience. If 'maleness' in this context was defined by the production of gametes via the male ejaculate, then the inability to produce fecundating sperm surely came as a striking blow to male identities (Inhorn 2004:169).

Here, the male gamete acts as an 'elaborating symbol' or a vehicle for ordering experience (Ortner 1973:1340). The presence of the male gamete, or sperm, defined and ordered the male body so that infertility, however 'temporary' it may be, disrupted things so that men were no longer able to position themselves in the 'natural order of things.' Infertility posed a threat not only to biological relations but also to their identity as constructed via socially recognised positions of husband-to-wife and father-to-child. The threat of infertility to the 'given' nature of this position, as part of their natural relational capacity considered to be inherent to the ontological status of being male, created an ontological uncertainty, which meant men needed to work at stabilising themselves relationally.

For most men in clinic, this meant undergoing extensive procedures so that their fertility might be recovered in the conception of a biologically related child. Most men discussed this process as a pursuit of 'natural' conception. Despite the highly technological processes involved in fertilisation, ART was perceived as the 'natural' way of doing things; bringing the male and female gametes together as was 'supposed' to happen 'naturally.' Simultaneously, men would invest in the social relations that stabilised them in the male roles of 'husband' and 'father.' This was particularly apparent in the way men emphasised how important it was to support their partners, even if this compromised their own endeavours to biologically reproduce, for example, if they decided to go ahead with IVF using donor sperm. In this, they played out what Thompson terms 'gender scripts' to perform overt and parodic hyper-gendered roles and situate themselves as relationally male (Thompson 2005:117–143). This meant that even if technologically assisted, biological fatherhood could not be achieved through clinical interventions, they could still assume the male role in the idealised family unit that was required for ART.[2]

The distinctions between the 'biological' and 'technical' and the 'biological' and 'social' allowed men to pursue masculinity in intersubjectively recognisable and validated ways. Clinical practice, the ultimate aim of which was producing children and therefore parents, entailed the coming together of things considered to be of different ontological orders: nature, society, technology, biology, male and female, sex and gender. Douglas (2002[1966]) maintains that systems of symbols are imperfect reflections of reality and that when the boundaries of taxonomy are broken or blurred, impurity emerges. Whilst being an 'infertile male' entailed a moment of identity crisis for many men, as they struggled to position themselves as not-producing the male gametes needed in order to conceive, the masculine positions of husband and father were still open to their pursuit. This was made capable only through the maintenance of carefully distinct categories that allowed them to use 'technology' to conceive 'naturally.' to adopt a 'social' role when the 'biological' one failed, and to maintain the 'gendered' performance of masculinity while no longer fitting the definition of a 'sexed' male. In this context, being an infertile man did not entail a hybridity, or coming together of orders of kinds, but a carefully staged ontological choreography that allowed for the pursuit of masculinity in its various forms.

This was not merely a symbolic process, but a material one. 'Male' and 'female' bodies were defined by their corporeal roles in reproduction and gender inequalities mapped onto these bodily differences. These positions

---

2 At this point, I want to clarify that all men attending clinic would be considered 'treatment seekers,' that is, they were all actively trying to conceive a biologically related child. In this, they were already actively engaging in the pursuit of being a father and/or a good partner in line with a particular understanding of what the male role is. It is important to recognise that this ethnography does not capture the multitude of ways in which identifying men may or may not perform their masculinities outside of this context; it does not attempt to draw conclusions about what it is 'to be male' more generally.

were product and productive of clinical practices: materialising in the hyper-medicalisation of the female body and the side-lining of the male. The active role the male body took in the production of the male ejaculate meant their reproductive role was not easily incorporated into medical control. The isolation of the male ejaculate outside the body in clinical space allowed for processes of diagnosis to be undertaken, as it came to perform in its own right. Removed from its usual situate and it was embedded in clearly defined and controlled parameters, stabilising its performance so that normal/abnormal could be identified and infertility determined. Functioning as a material synecdoche for male relational capacity, the contents of the male ejaculate revealed the 'truth' of the 'biological' ability to conceive. If this capacity was deemed to be subpar, then men could invest in the 'technological' and 'social' in order to stabilise themselves within male roles.

The ethnography presented here speaks against the emergence of 'new,' 'hybrid' kinds alongside ARTs. Presenting instead how in this context, human and natural kinds were kept distinct, their binaries used to reinforce each other, and their boundaries carefully maintained, through meticulously choreographed practices. This ontological choreography, moving in and around the material synecdoche of sperm, allowed men in clinic to pursue masculinity in a variety of ways but never so that they breached the boundary of being 'naturally' male – even if it needed to be achieved 'socially' of 'technologically.' Rather than mapping out an 'imperfect reality,' these systems of classification made up reality. The ethnography presented here demonstrates how this reality was performed in the RHU, constructing what it meant to be an infertile man in this context. The material analysis of clinical processes presented here demonstrates the ontological choreography undertaken to produce this position: a position made up of a natural, technological, biological, social, sexed, and gendered performance.

References

Becker, G. (2000). *The Elusive Embryo: How Women and Men Approach New Reproductive Technologies*. Berkeley: University of California Press.

Butler, J. (1990). *Gender Trouble: Feminism and the Subversion of Identity*. London: Routledge.

Butler, J. (1993). *Bodies that Matter: On the Discursive Limits of 'Sex'*. London: Routledge.

Carsten, J. (2001). Substantivism, Antisubstantivism, and Anti-antisubstantivism. In S. Franklin and S. McKinnon (Eds.), *Relative Values: Reconfiguring Kinship Studies*. Durham: Duke University Press, 29–54.

Culley, L., N. Hudson and M. Lohan (2013). Where are all the men? The marginalization of men in social scientific research on infertility. *Reproductive Biomedicine Online* 27:225–235.

Douglas, M. (2002 [1966]). *Purity and Danger: An Analysis of Concepts of Pollution and Taboo*. London: Psychology Press.

Dyer, S. J., N. Abrahams, et al. (2004). 'You are a Man Because you have Children': Experiences, reproductive health knowledge and treatment-seeking behaviour among men suffering from couple infertility in South Africa. *Human Reproduction* 19(4):960–967.

Fausto-Sterling, A. (1995). How to Build a Man. In M. Berger, B. Wallace and S. Watson (Eds.), *Constructing Masculinity*. London: Routledge, 127–135.

Foucault, M. (1995 [1975]). *Discipline & Punishment: The Birth of the Prison*. New York: Vintage Books.

Franklin, S. (2006). *Born and Made: An Ethnography of Pre-implantation Genetic Diagnosis*. Princeton: Princeton University Press.

Franklin, S. and S. Mckinnon (2001). Introduction. In S. Franklin and S. Mckinnon (Eds.), *Relative Values: Reconfiguring Kinship Studies*. Durham: Duke University Press, 1–25.

Goldberg, H. (2009). The Sex in the Sperm: Male Infertility and its Challenges to Masculinity in and Israeli-Jewish Context. In M. C. Inhorn, T. Tjørnhøj-Thomsen, H. Goldberg and M. la Cour Mosegaard (Eds.), *Reconceiving the Second Sex: Men, Masculinity and Reproduction*. New York: Berghahn, 203–225.

Hacking, I. (1995). The Looping Effects of Human Kinds. In D. Sperber, D. Premack and A. J. Premack (Eds.), *Causal Cognition: A Multidisciplinary Debate*. Oxford: Oxford University Press, 351–383.

Hudson, N. and L. Culley (2013). 'The bloke can be a bit hazy about what's going on': Men and cross-border reproductive treatment. *Reproductive Biomedicine Online* 27:253–260.

Human Fertilisation and Embryology Authority (2013). Fertility treatment 2011: Trends and figures. Accessed 19 April 2015. www.hfea.gov.uk/ivf-figures-2006.html.

Inhorn, M. (2004). Middle Eastern masculinities in the age of new reproductive technologies: Male infertility and stigma in Egypt and Lebanon. *Medical Anthropology Quarterly* 18(2):162–182.

Inhorn, M. (2012). *The New Arab Man: Emergent Masculinities, Technologies and Islam in the Middle East*. Princeton, NJ: Princeton University Press.

Katz, P. (1981). Ritual in the operating room. *Ethnology* 20(4):335–350.

Kleinman, A. (1980). *Patients and Healers in the Context of Culture*. Berkeley: University of California Press.

Knorr-Cetina, K. (1999). *Epistemic Cultures: How the Sciences Make Knowledge*. Cambridge, MA: Harvard University Press.

Latour, B. (1987). *Science in Action*. Cambridge, MA: Harvard University Press.

Latour, B. (1993 [1991]). *We Have Never Been Modern*. Trans. C. Porter. Cambridge, MA: Harvard University Press.

Lévi-Strauss, C. (1958). *Structural Anthropology*. London: Penguin Press.

Lupton, D. (1997). Foucault and the Medicalisation Critique. In A. Peterson and R. Bunton (Eds.), *Foucault, Health and Medicine*. London: Routledge, 94–110.

Lynch, M. (2017). *Art and Artifact in Laboratory Science (1985): A Study of Shop Work and Shop Talk in a Research Laboratory*. London: Routledge.

Martin, E. (1991). The egg and the sperm: How science has constructed a romance based on stereotypical male-female roles. *Signs* 16(3):485–501.

McCracken, G. (1989). Homeyness – A Cultural Account of one Constellation of Consumer Goods and Meaning. In E. Hirschman (Ed.), *Interpretive Consumer Research*. London: Association of Consumer Research, 168–183.

Mody, C. C. M. A. (2001). Little dirt never hurt anyone: Knowledge-making and contamination in materials science. *Social Studies of Science* 31(1):7–36.

Mol, A. (2000). Pathology and the Clinic: An Ethnographic Presentation of two Atheroscleroses. In M. Lock, A. Young and A. Cambrosio (Eds.), *Living and Working with the New Medical Technologies: Intersections of Enquiry*. Cambridge: Cambridge University Press, 82–102.

Morgan, L. H. (1871). *Systems of Consanguinity and Affinity of the Human Family*. Washington: Smithsonian Institution Press.

Muller, J. H. (1994). Anthropology, bioethics, and medicine: A provocative trilogy. *Medical Anthropology Quarterly* 8(4):448–467.

OED (2015). *Online version*. Fordham University Library Database.

Ortner, S. (1974). Is Female to Male as Nature is to Culture? In M. Rosaldo and L. Lamphere (Eds.), *Women, Culture and Society*. Stanford: Stanford University Press, 67–88.

Pedersen, M. A. (2012). Common nonsense: A review of certain recent reviews on the 'Ontological Turn'. *Anthropology of This Century* 5. Accessed 12 February 2015. http://aotcpress.com/articles/common_nonsense/.

Rawlings, B. (1989). Coming clean: The symbolic use of clinical hygiene in a hospital sterilising unit. *Sociology of Health & Illness* 11(3):279–293.

Strathern, M. (1992). *After Nature: English Kinship in the Late Twentieth Century*. Cambridge: Cambridge University Press.

Thompson, C. (2005). *Making Parents: The Ontological Choreography of Reproductive Technologies*. Cambridge, MA: MIT Press.

Tilley, C. (1997). *A Phenomenology of Landscape: Places, Paths and Monuments*. Oxford: Berg.

Waitzkin, H. (1984). Doctor-patient communication: Clinical implications of social scientific research. *Jama* 252(17):2441–2446.

Zegers-Hochschild, F., G. D. Adamson, J. de Mouzon, O. Ishihara, R. Mansour, K. Nygren, E. Sullivan and S. Van der Poel (2009). The international committee for monitoring assisted reproductive technology (ICMART) and the world health organization (WHO) revised glossary on ART terminology, 2009. *Human Reproduction* 24(11):2683–2687.

Part II
Infrastructures of care

6 Blood, lungs, and passports

Aaron Parkhurst

Introduction

This chapter explores the material conditions of residence in Dubai and other Arabian Gulf states, showing how they are inexorably tied to the materials of health-screening processes (x-rays and vials of blood for TB and HIV, respectively). These medical materials, due to their nature, are a microcosm of both the physical and social body and person. They are also locally known as potent symbols of the body and dirt, informing the ways in which people understand health and purity in relation to the human body. This ethnography follows migrant men as they participate in residential health-screening and navigate these medical materialities to develop a highly sought-after form of social and political legitimacy in personhood. Migrant men in Dubai are highly aware of their precarious position. They are made subject to human rights abuses, but they often have their own motivations in making themselves subject to these regimes. Failed medical testing results in immediate deportation from the country, and these men are not given the results of their tests. In this regard, migrants are made subject to processes of biopolitics that construct notions of cleanliness and dirtiness through bureaucratic medical hegemony.

The narratives presented in this chapter both begin and end not at the clinic, or the workplace, but at the airport. It could begin elsewhere – in Kerala province where men cannot find work to support their families, in towns and cities in Sri Lanka or rural Nepal where political and infrastructural collapse has forced young men to seek the means to survive elsewhere, or throughout the Philippines, where the promise of employment, cash, and a bit of glamour have motivated both men and women in equal measure to migrate to the Arabian Peninsula. The background and motivations of the migrants who come to the Arabian Gulf matter. The decision to come to Dubai, Abu Dhabi, Riyadh, Doha, Bahrain, or any of the other rapidly growing cosmopolitan places of the Gulf is rarely taken lightly. In many cases, it might not be best understood as a 'decision' at all, as the conditions of society force migrants into systems of labour in which debates on agency are more academic than practised. Ethnography, such as Alice

Elliot's research among Moroccan migrants, and the wives and family left behind, has shown how these paradigms of migration have radically shaped those societies from which people emigrate, complicating traditional forms of kinship, love, and relationships, and even profoundly shaping identity and subjectivity among those who 'wait' to emigrate (Elliot 2016; Elliot et al. 2017). The narratives could also end elsewhere, in the places some migrants return to, permanently, seasonally, or for short visits. Ethnography has shown how systems of migration and return to Sri Lanka from the Gulf, for example, have reframed gender relations and constructs of well-being, and have often challenged the very moral structures of Sri Lankan life (Ally 2014). The narratives in this chapter, however, begin and end at the airport in Dubai, where migrants carry with them and embody these paradigms of hope and hype, success and failure.

The narratives also begin, here, with the loss of a personal object – a small book, made mostly of paper, used during travel for identification. Migrants arrive at the international terminal in Dubai, or more cheaply, in neighbouring Sharjah, in large groups. They are recruited in their home countries by contractors for large development firms, or retail chains, or through word of mouth about catering positions. They need a government-issued passport in order to travel, and, for most workers, this document is expensive. Those migrants who might come to Dubai to work in development, as cheap labour to build the rapidly growing city, are often chaperoned during travel, or they are met in large groups at the airport by representatives of their employment. Their passports are confiscated before they reach customs. The chaperone approaches the customs agent with all the passports, together with copies of contracts. The agent compares the passports to the contracts and allows the group into the country. The migrants are then bussed, without their passport, to their accommodation, in worker camps, or perhaps in shared housing elsewhere in the desert. Dubai customs is their first administrative hurdle upon entering the country. Their passport takes the place of their person. Their next bureaucratic experience will be their medical screening.

Prominent thinkers within Material Culture Studies have asked scholars to know systems of social relations by 'following the object' as a methodological imperative (Myers 2001; Appadurai 1986). Appadurai suggests that ethnographically following objects of study creates an epistemology that is foreign to most areas of science – that objects are best understood as having social lives themselves. Knowing these social lives highlights, in turn, the social lives of men and women whose relationships inform, and are informed by the objects they make, love, use, discard, or need in exotic, mundane, or quotidian purpose. In accordance, Nicholas Thomas stresses that the fluid and dynamic nature of culture, its changing biases and assumptions, are just as evident in the social lives of things as they are in humans, even when the physical form of these 'things' remain static (1991). It is clear, then, that the history of the thing matters (Thomas 1991) or, as Kopytoff has argued, its biography (1986). These methodologies have been critiqued, however, as simply creating signifiers of human lives. As Pinney has argued,

> The fate of objects . . . is always to live out the social life of men, or to become entangled in the webs of culture whose ability to refigure the object simultaneously inscribes culture's ability to translate things into signs and the object's powerlessness as an artifactual trace. Narratives of the social lives of things, they reaffirm the agency of those humans they pass between.
>
> (Pinney 2005:259)

Pinney, in his critiques of materiality, asks the social scientist to be wary of circularity, and search instead for 'jolts and disjunctions' (2005:270). I suggest that migrant passports in Dubai might afford one such disjunction. Indeed, 'following the object,' as Myers or Appadurai ask one to, can take one only so far in this context. The passports are taken at the airport, but they are not returned to their owners. They are passed on to their employers who sponsor their workers' residency. It can, of course, be observed that politics, socialities, and identity are embedded in the object. Governments deny people the right to free travel, only to sell it back to them. Freedom of movement is contingent upon the physical presence of these small paper books. The business owners who confiscate passports create powerful systems of hegemony through the use of the object. Workers' rights, their living conditions, their salaries, and their work safety are unable to be negotiated when employees lack the fundamental right to walk away. One can argue that the passport is a material nexus of these politics, or perhaps it is better to say that these conditions are best highlighted in its absence, rather than in the object itself. In any case, following the social life of the passport would prove a dead end for social scientists researching the lives of migrants in Dubai. The passports are taken and kept in a safe. They are pulled out once every two years, when Dubai labour law affords migrants a trip to their home countries. Their materiality might, following Pinney's call, best be understood as a disjuncture. I argue that the affective affordances of the passport are tied to the materials and processes used and performed in medical screenings. What follows is, first, an account of these screening processes, as experienced by myself and my interlocutors at a large screening hospital facility in Deira neighbourhood in Dubai. This is followed by brief stories of young migrants, and their experience with medical screenings that illustrate the relationships between people, their bodies, blood and lungs, their passports, and their perceived future.

Deira hospital

At the time of research between 2007 and 2010, all immigrants to Dubai, regardless of their country of origin, are required to have medical screening for their work or residency permits. Not all visitors to Dubai are required to have these screenings, as not all visitors require visas to enter the country. Visitors from select countries are allowed entry to the UAE without a visa, though these visitors are expected to be short-term visitors. When work or residency permits are successful, medical tests must be re-administered every two years. In September of 2008, I drove myself and four migrant workers, all young men, to a large medical screening facility in Deira, on the north side of Dubai's Creek, to obtain the blood work and x-ray screenings necessary for residence visas in Dubai. We were meeting three others at the facility, as they lived nearby and could make their own way there. I was responsible for all of our paperwork. The eight of us migrated to Dubai from four nations. I came to Dubai as a researcher from the UK, applying for a work permit on an American passport. Three of the young men had migrated from the Philippines, three had recently arrived from Sri Lanka, and one from Nepal. In terms of the consequences for a failed medical screening, our nationalities were irrelevant. Any failed medical screening results in eventual deportation. For most, this deportation would be immediate. As mentioned, hired labour in the development industry, or in the catering industry, and often in retail, are recruited abroad. The company that hires and sponsors the employee pays for the flight to Dubai, funds short-term housing, pays residence visa fees and pays for medical screening. The screenings are testing for a range of conditions, including pregnancy, Hepatitis, Syphilis, Leprosy, HIV/AIDS, and Tuberculosis (TB). Aside from pregnancy tests, any condition that tested positive resulted in immediate deportation. Depending on the severity of the condition, immigrants may first be quarantined while they await the return of their passports for travel back to their home country. Pregnancy does not result in forced deportation, but employers are informed and allowed to terminate the contract. Depending on the nature of employment (maids, retail, or catering, for example), these women are likely to be expelled from the country, as it is illegal for many women to remain in the UAE without company sponsorship. The pregnancy test carries other risks as well. It is illegal to have sex outside of marriage in the UAE. Each of the seven Emirates has their own terms of enforcement and understanding of extra-marital sex, with some more liberal than others. Nonetheless, the risk remains in each Emirate that a pregnant woman who cannot prove she is married can be arrested for extra-marital sex, imprisoned, or deported on these grounds. This chapter, however, is primarily concerned with the screenings for HIV and Tuberculosis, which require blood samples and x-rays, respectively.

The hospital screening facility that we were visiting is primarily for large groups of male migrant workers. Women did not attend this facility. Thousands of people require medical fitness tests each day. This hospital, and another facility in nearby Satwa, are notoriously busy, overcrowded, and chaotic, and the waiting times stretch for many hours – and sometimes into several days (see Dhal and Hilotin 2011, for example). They are, however, inexpensive. Expatriates from 'Western' countries are unlikely to be waiting at these facilities. Companies that hire professionals from Europe or North America, for example, are well aware of the chaos and uncomfortableness of these facilities, and often pay decent money for their employees to be screened elsewhere in the city. Employers for migrant workers from other countries, however, are not willing to pay the fees. This may be why, despite widespread acknowledgement that screening infrastructure has been very poor for several decades, little progress has been made. Visitors to the region with the privilege to complain are able to get their tests in more sanitary conditions in which patients wait only several minutes at pre-booked appointments. It is one of the many bureaucratic processes that separate visitors to the country into divergent categories of 'expats' and 'migrants' (for a broader discussion of these categories, see Steegar 2009, or Fedorak 2017:152).

The hospital in Deira will process the medical tests for any men, but the assumption is that it is designed to process "migrant" men. We arrived at 8:30 a.m., handed our paperwork to receptionists and then collected our numbers. The hospital calls groups in sets of 20–25 at a time, and we knew we had several hours at least. We attempt to find space in the waiting room. There are several areas where people await their screening. The first is closest to the actual tests. It is a small space with room to seat about 20 people, though there are roughly a hundred in the room. This area is where people wait once their sets of numbers have been called, and the men have self-organised themselves into queues. The second and largest is akin to a mid-sized warehouse. There are benches and chairs lined throughout, and hundreds of men, mostly from the Indian subcontinent, dressed in mundu or light grey trousers, sit cramped together across the room. There are a few small televisions in the corner, showing daytime soap operas in Hindi or Malayalam, and they are subtitled in a script I cannot read. The room is surprisingly quiet, aside from the noise of industrial fans attempting to circulate air. There are several faucets for water, and there is a small queue for each of them.

The outside of the hospital has strips of plants, dirt, and grass lined with date palms – likely planted some generations ago. There is the noise of crowded Deira all around, and this part of the city is hotter than some others. The palms offer little shade, but the strikingly beautiful red branches of nearby Gulmohar trees offer far more. These are often prime property throughout the city for workers as they escape the oppressive sun. Here, they lay on top of each other holding each other's hands, as they do elsewhere in the city while they relax, waiting for their testing. It is far more pleasant outside than in, if one can tolerate the sun. We sit outside for several hours and picnic, waiting for our series of numbers to be called. The Filipino men have been through this process before, and they have brought card games and music. The rest are new to the country, and they all use the time to get to know each other. They talk about their families back home, movies they may have seen, and pop music. They also talk about medicine. The South Asian men want to know if the blood test or the x-ray hurts. They have heard that it does. They have heard that the doctor takes too much blood, but they do not have a volume to compare to. They are surprised to hear that the results of the tests usually take several weeks. They had heard that one is arrested at the hospital if one is sick, and that one is then put in jail. They also ask me why I have to be tested, as 'people coming from London don't have to be tested.' I explain that this is mandatory for everyone, but I'm not sure they believe me. They tell me they had assumed I came because they needed a chaperone.

Members of the group have different conceptions of what they are tested for. The men from the Philippines speak English well, and use named categories of illness – HIV and TB. Others talk about vague sickness, independent of their level of English. They speak in the same terms as many in England and the US – that as being 'clean,' or 'not clean' – terms of engagement that I will refer to later. They are afraid of going to prison in general. There is a mystery among the population regarding Dubai laws, and what is illegal or not. For example, my Filipino colleagues have brought their own lunch to the hospital – pork sausages and rice. Pork can be bought at most grocery stores in sections with large signs that read 'No Muslims Allowed.' Products with pork in them can also be sold at many licenced restaurants. Yet my colleagues are not sure if and where they can consume pork, and they always feel that they need to be clever when eating their lunch. Many of them consume alcohol as well, though they do not have the required special alcohol licence to purchase alcoholic beverages. They talk about going to prison for being sick, but most are worried about something they feel is worse – being sent home. The workers from South Asia avoid speaking in terms of deportation. Rather, they refer to their passports. 'They gave him back his passport' becomes a way to refer to the failure to immigrate.

It can be a celebratory statement as well. A man whom I befriended in my four years in Dubai proudly announced to me that after 23 years he was getting his passport back. He was a cleaner in one of Sheikh Zayed Road's skyscrapers and had been a cleaner in the city under different contracts for over two decades. His documents would have been pulled regularly over these years, for several trips back home to Kerala to see his wife and children, for new medical screenings under different employers, or for general renewal. Nonetheless, he beamed with pride as he announced his retirement through his documents. I suspect he cared little for the material thing; his pride was in having earned the possibility to return to his green country and stay with his family long term. Still, the document has his name and likeness printed in its pages, a likeness that was miniaturised and placed in a security safe for the most part of 23 years. The passport's materiality affords an inalienability. Written on the document is a warning that one should always keep the passport in one's own possession, and it is often insisted upon by most foreign missions. It is, according to UAE law since 2002, illegal for employers to hold on to passports any longer than is necessary to obtain visas, yet it remains common practice for employers to confiscate them. Like the inalienable possessions written in Annette Weiner's famous interpretations of object exchange in Papua New Guinea and Samoa (1992), these passports are able to construct and rebalance powerful forms of social hierarchy in their exchange. However, unlike the objects (and women) of exchange in Weiner's analysis, these goods are not in any way gifts given but, rather, inalienable goods taken. Hierarchies are defeated only when the good is returned to its owner.

However, my friend is able to receive his document in the personal knowledge that his migrant experience has succeeded in ways in which he can relate. He has spent many years sending money home to his wife and children, who are grown themselves. He is returning home with a narrative of fulfiling the promises to which migration to the Gulf often speaks. My friend succeeded, but I suggest his passport also served as a material success. I argue that my interlocutors at the hospital are so preoccupied with their documents because of the passport's potential as a material failure. This is, as we have argued elsewhere, 'to suggest that in the individual subject's (or collective societal) project of inscribing themselves in the world, failure happens when the material and social stuff of that inscription behaves in ways other than intended' (Carroll et al. 2017:2). When it is returned early, through redundancy, or a failed medical screening, the passport works as intended as a document of identification and travel, but in important ways it fails to work socially in the ways in which it promises. The moral imperatives that inspired men and women to leave their homelands become instantly arrested. When medical tests fail, the inalienability of the passports become highlighted in new ways; they become intimately entwined with the human body.

Six hours pass. After lunch, the afternoon sun becomes too much to bear. The large waiting room has become slightly less crowded, and the hot humidity requires that we move indoors. The friendliness and energy that characterised the morning turns into boredom. Hours pass and hundreds more migrant workers are processed through the test centre. At 6:00 p.m., I find some fast food across the street, and as the sun is beginning to set, we go back outside. The desert air is at its best just after the sun sets. Escaping the hospital lifts my friends' spirits. We chat for several hours, and around 8:30 p.m., our block of numbers is called. Several of the men grow suddenly silent and their faces turn white. We enter the small waiting room and join the makeshift lines. There is still some time to go as the 'real' queue begins in the hallways after the waiting room. As we approach the halls, my friends chat about medicine, doctors, and what happened the last time they were tested. The men from South Asia ask again for the experiences of the Filipino men, who have been here before. We enter the hallway, and the queue becomes deadly silent. There is still 20 minutes to wait, and no one speaks.

The x-ray comes first. Men are called by their numbers five or six at a time, and they remove their shirts. Their forms are handed to a technician who stands them, one by one, in the machine. The men are nervous, but the test does not take long. It is a quick scan, examining the lungs for scar tissue as a result of TB. If the test comes back positive, the workers are banned from the country for life. The rates of TB in the country are very low, with only two cases per 100,000 persons, but according to the Health Authority of Abu Dhabi (2017), this is because of successful screens, as the incidence of TB for new arrivals to the country is 20 times higher than the local populace. The x-ray is designed to screen for both active TB and scars that show old cases. At the time of research, both resulted in deportation. However, the tests have some limitations and failures. There are a number of other conditions, some of which are quickly treatable, that can show up as positive results during the screening. Some of the men are fascinated by the medical technology but are unable to see their x-ray images. As each man finishes his scan, he moves towards the corner of the room. The men huddle together until the group is finished. When the last of the set of numbers are finished, the men put their shirts back on and move to a new hallway to wait for their blood to be taken. The x-ray images are not processed immediately. After several days, technicians will review the scan and return the results to the employer or sponsor. If the images show scars, a person might be called in for a second test for clarity.

The men are led into a new queue in an adjoining hallway. There is only a very short wait, as the process is more controlled now that the men are in a more clinical space. The wait for the x-ray had made the men nervous, but not as much as the blood samples, and they do not speak to each other. There are four clinicians taking blood samples, and they work simultaneously at different desks in a moderately sized space. The men are called over to the desks by number. The clinicians are also from South Asia and some are able to communicate in a language in which some of the men are more comfortable. The men are asked from which arm they would like their blood taken, though some do not understand the question. The men are shaking, and the clinicians have to remind them many times to hold still. The migrant workers are encouraged to look away. The clinician rubs antiseptic on the bicep, and they inject a needle into the arm. In most cases, the blood flows easily. The process takes 30 seconds.

'Blood,' as a bodily substance, has been one of the most scrutinised material goods in anthropology. There is not space here to cover its social significance in the depth that it warrants. A quick review shows that it has been understood by foundational thinkers in anthropology as being the very 'stuff' of kinship (Sahlins 2011), but it also highlights both class and race (Weston 2001). It is the material metaphor for life itself in many Judeo-Christian practices (borrowing from Leviticus 17:11) and is used as a substance of devotion in modern Hinduism (Copeman 2009). Other prominent anthropologists have suggested that human social preoccupation with blood is the very origin of culture: where its simultaneous taboo and reverence in the social engagement with menstruation highlight blood as the natural symbol of sex and fertility (Knight 1991); where its biologically cyclical patterns afford the potential for people to understand themselves, to borrow the language of Bourdieu, as 'scanned in the rhythms of nature' (Bourdieu 1963:57). As Janet Carsten writes in her review of 'blood in context' across anthropology,

> Blood may be particularly apt for . . . metaphorical extension because it scores so highly in all three respects: It is visually striking, it can be seen inside and outside the body – both routinely and in exceptionally dramatic circumstances – and it can be obviously associated with life or life's cessation. The example of blood also underlines how these three different aspects are, in fact, inseparable and reinforce each other.
>
> (Carsten 2011:24)

The importance of blood as material culture cannot be stressed enough, and because blood can be all these things at once, it is difficult to scrutinise fully, here, the complexity of engagements my interlocutors have with this blood at the medical test centres. They are asked to flex their arms, and they can see the blood flowing in their veins. They can watch as the red fluid leaves their body, as it is collected by a stranger in a foreign place, attached to a label and some forms, and sent away. This can mean many different things to different people. When Mary Douglas published her now-famous monograph on *Natural Symbols* in 1970, blood was at the core of her attention. I suggest that blood's profound materiality is embedded, then, in her assertion that it provides a 'natural system of symbolising' (1970:xxxiii). The analysis in this chapter explores only one aspect of this materiality – and it is related to another of Douglas' contributions to Anthropology, that of a framework to think through cleanliness and dirt (1966). Like the passports, the blood, too, is inalienable from the person from which it is taken, and this inalienability helps inform the material disjunctures between bodily substance and travel document. They are tied to each other, and to the immigrant, through constructs of 'dirt.' The men are distinctly aware that a stranger, and eventually the state, now has their blood. They are aware as well that their employer will have access to the results in some way. They are profoundly cognisant that their personhood will be judged upon the status of their blood as 'clean.'

After the blood test, the men are free to leave the centre. They pile silently into my jeep, and I drive them home to their accommodation in Satwa. They do not speak a word on the way home. This is partly due to exhaustion. It is after 10 p.m. and the intensely humid desert air has taken its toll on their bodies. The length of the day at the centre makes the testing experience physically demanding. The nature of the testing is also psychologically and emotionally exhausting. They have felt an embodied nervousness for many hours. When the day is over, they cannot go home with the exuberance of a large stress being lifted. The results of these tests are still pending, and their emotions are left unresolved. Over the next few days, the men repeatedly ask me if I've heard about the results of their screenings. I explain that I will never have access to that information, but they continue to ask nonetheless. The new migrants to Dubai began working the day after they arrived, several weeks before their medical tests, and they continue to work full time while they wait for the results. They receive their first paycheck, though the employer manages their bank accounts, and so rent and other fees are automatically deducted. This is a common policy, and the employers claim that it is in the best interest of the workers. Many forms of debt in the Emirates are illegal, and so the practice does protect workers from draconian policy. However, employers in Dubai are legally responsible for the movements and actions of their employees, and controlling their accounts, like their passports, is a way to control their movement through the city. Many employees simply do not trust their workers, but the migrants with whom I spoke claimed to prefer the system. They made so little, and it made their lives easier.

Waiting and results

After two weeks of waiting, I grew impatient. I need my passport to travel to Oman, and it had not yet been returned to me. I contacted the head offices, and when they discovered my nationality, my passport was returned to me within a day. I enquired on the results of the screenings for the men I had accompanied, but they explained it was not their policy to share that information. In the end, all of the men I accompanied to the health centre passed their medical screenings, but they were never informed. After several weeks, the men from South Asia began asking more regularly. The Filipino workers who had been through this system before explained '[The result] only takes a few days, just as long as you don't get your passport back . . . everything is fine for this. Don't be worried.' As more time passed, the men became confident that their lungs and their blood had been judged clean enough to remain in the country. They say, relieved, 'I don't think they will be giving it back to us.' However, while they waited, the tension was exacerbated by the results of another employee.

A young Filipina migrant woman who had been working as their colleague for two months had undergone the screening on the same day as the men, but at another hospital better suited for women. Several weeks after the tests, she was called to an office where she was told she would need to leave the country. By law, the employer is responsible for arranging flights back to the Philippines with haste, and the young woman was given 12 hours' notice to collect her things and say goodbye to the people she had befriended. The company would drive her directly to the airport. Her colleagues were shaken and upset, though many had seen this happen before to others. They never spoke of her deportation directly. As mentioned at the beginning of this chapter, they instead refer to the travel documents. They explain, 'They gave her her passport. She had to have her passport, and *fwoosh.*' They make a hand gesture of a plane taking off. They know she had failed her medical screening. The young woman herself did not know why she failed. The parent company did not give her the results; they simply returned her travel documents. The direct employers were, I believe, genuinely worried for her, and they tried to help her organise tests for when she returned to the Philippines to learn more about her health, but they were also irritated that they had spent nearly two months training a new employee, including the financial costs of her flights to and from the country. Some of her compatriots, however, were heartbroken. None of them, to my knowledge, knew the true nature of the woman's health, but when they spoke of the passport, they also spoke of her lungs. The assumption was that she failed the x-ray. HIV/AIDS was not an option. The stigmatisation for the condition is still so prevalent in the region that it is very rare to hear it spoken of openly. A problem of the lungs for these migrant men and women is a failure to migrate and, as discussed previously, this has moral implications. However, just as Susan Sontag has famously written in other contexts (1989), a failure of their blood is, for them, a moral failure in itself. In any case, as mentioned in the chapter's introduction, her narrative ends in this chapter at the airport. The employer (or recruitment company) organises her check-in and chaperones her to security. She is then handed her passport, and the chaperone watches to make sure she has exited the country. Her body, her health, her lungs, her blood, and her pocket-sized passport are now, in some regard, materially and socially reunited. Without the results of the screening, the failure of her migration, and everything this failure implies, is materially configured within her travel documents.

Conclusion

I set about in this chapter to illustrate how the successes and failures of migration can be understood through a disjuncture of the material goods of migration processes. I am not arguing that blood, lungs, and passports are best understood as metaphorically or socially synonymous. Rather, for new migrants, the failures of blood, lungs, and personhood to cohere within the medical screenings in Dubai is made clear through the presence of the passport. They are united in that they afford an inalienability of the object to the person. For the anthropologist, this makes following their disjuncture, rather than simply following the objects themselves, ethnographically possible. They are also united in a system of symbolising – that of dirt. The screenings highlight a salient condition of migrant personhood in Dubai. That is, migrants are 'dirty' until proven clean. They watch as 'expats' and tourists from select countries are able to enter the country and move freely. These groups are 'clean' until proven dirty. The men with whom I spent my hours at the clinic, and with whom I spent many months after, were able to work and live in the country after their screening. The success of their blood and lungs was articulated and made coherent though their passport's invisibility. They have the ability to stay resident in the country, and many can use their wages to support their families in their home countries, but they have given up their right to free movement, and while I have not the space to discuss it here, they have given up other rights as well. The next time they see their travel documents will be in two years' time, at the airport, when Dubai law requires that employers allow a vacation back home for migrants to see their families. They will return to work after a month. Their passports will be again be confiscated, and they will be due for health-screening renewal. I add, as a final point, that many of my informants in my years in the Emirates have their own distinction between 'expats' and migrants. In discussing the two categories, they speak of wealth, or nationality, and even of skin colour, but most saliently and most commonly, they speak of passports. They know that expats hold their own, and migrants do not. Examining, then, the 'jolts and disjunctures' of the object may, indeed, uncover affective affordances that speak to much larger structures of society, politics, and personhood beyond health and the body.

References

Ally, S. (2014). 'Good Women Stay at Home. Bad Women Go Everywhere': Agency, Sexuality and Self in Sri Lankan Migrant Narratives. In Sunil K. Khanna and Maya Unnithan-Kumar (Eds.), *The Cultural Politics of Reproduction: Migration, Health and Family Making*. London: Berghahn Books, 50–76.

Appadurai, A. (Ed.) (1986). *Social Life of Things: Commodities in Cultural Perspective*. Cambridge: Cambridge University Press.

Bourdieu, P. (1963). The Attitude of the Algerian Peasant toward Time. In J. Pitt-Rivers (Ed.), *Mediterranean Countrymen: Essays in the Social Anthropology of the Mediterranean*. Paris: Mouton, 55–72.

Carroll, T., D. Jeevendrampillai and A. Parkhurst (2017). Introduction: Toward a general theory of failure. In Carroll et al. (Eds.), *Material Culture of Failure: When Things Do Wrong*. London: Bloomsbury, 1–20.

Carsten, J. (2011). Substance and relationality: Blood in contexts. *Annual Review of Anthropology* 40:19–35.

Copeman J. (2009). *Veins of Devotion: Blood Donation and Religious Experience in North India*. New Brunswick, NJ/London: Rutgers University Press.

Dhal, S. and J. Hilotin (2011). Tests that test your patience. *Gulf News* 2 June 2011. Accessed 4 February 2018. http://gulfnews.com/leisure/health/tests-that-test-your-patience-1.816374.

Douglas, M. (1966). *Purity and Danger* (Vol. 68). London: Routledge.

Douglas, M. (1970). *Natural Symbols* (1996 ed.). London: Routledge.

Elliot, A. (2016). Paused subjects: Waiting for migration in North Africa. *Time & Society* 25(1):102–116. ISSN 0961–463X

Elliot, A., R. Norum, and N. Salazar (Eds.) (2017). *Methodologies of Mobility: Ethnography and Experiment*. New York: Berghahn. ISBN 978-1-78533-480-1.

Fedorak, S. (2017). *Anthropology Matters: Third Edition*. Toronto: University of Toronto Press.

Kopytoff, I. (1986). The Cultural Biography of Things: Commoditization as Process. In Appadurai (Ed.), *Social Life of Things: Commodities in Cultural Perspective*. Cambridge: Cambridge University Press, 64–93.

Knight C. (1991). *Blood Relations: Menstruation and the Origin of Culture*. New Haven, CT: Yale University Press.

Myers, F. (2001). The Empire of Things: Regimes of Value and Material Culture. In *Advanced Seminar Series. School of American Research Advanced Seminar Series*. School of American Research Press.

Pinney, C. (2005). *Things Happen: Or, From Which Moment Does that Object Come? In: Materiality*. Duke University Press Books.

Sahlins M. (2011). What kinship is (part one). *Journal of the Royal Anthropological Institute* 17(1):2–19.

Sontag, S. (1989). *AIDS and Its Metaphors*. New York: Farrar, Straus and Giroux.

Steegar, S. (2009). *Cultures of Mobility: New Global Nomadism, Third Culture, and the Influence of Study Abroad*. Saarbruken: VDM Verlag Dr. Müller.

Thomas, N. (1991). *Entangled Objects: Exchange, Material Culture, and Colonialism in the Pacific*. Cambridge: Harvard University Press.

Weiner, A. (1992). *Inalienable Possessions: The Paradox of Keeping-while-giving*. Berkeley: University of California Press.

Weston, K. (2001). Kinship, Controversy, and the Sharing of Substance: The Race/class Politics of Blood Transfusion. See Franklin & McKinnon 2001, 147–174.

7 'Time for tea'

Tea practices and care in a British hospice

Sophie Duckworth

This chapter explores tea practices in the context of a British hospice as a service of care, as material affordances for emotional care, and as a symbolic artefact in the modern-day death ritual. Following a brief introduction to tea-drinking practices, tracing its history into the hospice movement, I introduce my ethnographic research in a British hospice that led me to explore the meanings of tea-drinking practices in the context of hospice care.

'Tea began as a medicine and grew into a beverage' (Okakura 1906:1). Tea was reportedly first drank in China in the fifth century and brought to Britain only during the seventeenth century. Complex historical and social contexts have influenced and helped create various tea-drinking practices in Britain over time. Tea-drinking practices are now so firmly embedded into various aspects of British culture that there is an apparent 'unconscious view' that tea drinking is a 'normal thing' (Farrell 2002:297). There is also a 'ceremony and ritual surrounding the institution of tea' that is seen to 'fulfil social needs' (ibid). It forms part of a habituated daily routine for many people. It is experienced as a comfort. It is a gesture of hospitality and sociality, but it has also been imbued with many other abstract therapeutic benefits such that it is seen as a 'a cure-all for life's ills' (Golby 2015). Scientists have also used empirical tests in order to demonstrate the therapeutic physiological effects of the beverage. It is thought that caffeine and thiamine, found in black tea, may help with alertness and improve mood by working on neurotransmitters in the brain (Quinlan et al. 1997; Quinlan et al. 2000; Einöther and Martens 2013; Sharangi 2009). The physical warmth of tea is often described as a 'comfort,' and it is thought that when offering another person a cup of tea, one might associate feelings of interpersonal warmth such as 'kindness' and 'trust' (Williams and Bargh 2008). Tea drinking is largely regarded as a social and psychological phenomenon (Verma 2013). This warmth and its associated notions of kindness and trust are, I found, linked for many to notions of 'home,' such that the material warmth of tea fosters feelings of comfort and nurturance. Whilst many have tried to document their own recipes and 'golden rules' for creating the perfect cup of tea (e.g. Orwell 1946), a 'cup of tea' is subject to personal preference and praxis and can materialise to be a variety of warm, ochre-coloured beverages served in any sort of vessel. Tea is, then, both general and medicinal and highly subjective and interpersonal.

'Modern' British hospices emerged from the late 1960s following Dame Cicely Saunders' 'Hospice movement' in London. At the time, death was perceived to be overly 'medicalised' (Illich 1976), and hospitals failed to provide adequate care for the dying. Pioneers of the hospice movement argued that death had come to be seen as a medical failure, whereas it should be seen as a normal part of life (Twycross 1992:6). The movement placed an emphasis on 'care' rather than 'cure,' arguing for less medical intervention and more supportive care for both the patient and the family, allowing them to 'live until you die' (Munley 1983:35; DuBois 1980:73–4). Saunders developed the notion of 'total pain,' aiming to provide a holistic framework in which to provide care for dying patients that purposefully contrasted the objectifying nature of common hospital settings (O'Brien 1993). Hospices were both intended and interpreted as homely, congenial spaces to welcome the dying patients and their families; Cicely Saunders spoke of the ideals of hospices being 'the kind of family and home that can give the welcome and hospitality of a good home' (Saunders 1965).

The term 'hospice' now refers to a 'concept of care' rather than a physical space (Clemens et al. 2003) and much of the 'care' is provided in patients' homes rather than in a hospice building, yet there remains the perception amongst many that hospices are places 'where people come to die' (Martin 2014). Over the years, the role of hospices has expanded to provide supportive care for patients with cancer and non-cancer-related terminal illnesses at any point along the disease trajectory, not just at the end of life. Whilst most hospices began as independent charitable organisations relying on voluntary donations and on volunteers for their operation, this became unsustainable and, consequently, most hospices became, at least in part, reliant on the government for some of their funding. While private hospices still exist in the British context, hospice care has been fully incorporated under the jurisdiction of the National Health Service.

As a medical student, I recall sitting with a palliative care consultant for the morning's clinic in a hospice. Whilst in the waiting area outside, every patient and their relatives would be offered a cup of tea, which they then brought into the clinic consultation with them. We all sat in the clinic room: the consultant, the patient, relative, and myself with our cups of tea. An emotive discussion ensued around the patient's terminal diagnosis and the shift from curative treatment to that of palliative hospice care. I remember reflecting, as I sat in the room, on the situation and how it came to pass. I became aware of the warm cups of tea in our hands; we sat together in silence punctuated only by sipping. I was not sure why, but I felt somehow that, at that moment in time, those cups of tea were important. This experience, and countless similar experiences within healthcare, have been the stimulus for this research investigating tea practices within a British hospice.

End-of-life care and 'hospice care' is something that I have become familiar with in the context of my work over the course of ten years leading up to this fieldwork. I have worked in both hospices and hospitals in England and Wales in a caring role, as a healthcare assistant,[1] and in a medical capacity during my years in training and practicing as a doctor. Within these roles, I have been regularly present at the death of patients and routinely needed to communicate with bereaved relatives. Furthermore, I have found myself serving tea in such situations out of a tacit, formerly unquestioned, but personal sense of 'care' for patients. I have often witnessed a positive affect from offering tea to patients and their relatives in times when I felt there was little else I could offer.

This chapter is based on an ethnographic study conducted in a British hospice during the year of 2016. This involved participant observation in the hospice building alongside semi-structured interviews with healthcare staff such as nurses, doctors, domiciliary workers, and volunteers. Fieldwork was predominantly focused on an inpatient ward in the hospice; however, I found that tea practices were present all over the hospice, with tea-making facilities in almost every room. The moment one walked through the doors of the hospice there was the 'tea bar' run by volunteers who considered themselves the 'welcoming committee.' On the ward, patients would typically stay for anything from a few days to a couple of weeks for the assessment and management of their symptoms and then discharged back home or to their place of care but some also remained in the hospice for their last days of life. It soon became apparent that tea practices were fully embedded into practices of care within the hospice, serving patients both physical and emotional support.

'Care,' as will become apparent, is a polythetic term. It describes, on one hand, a practical 'service of care' such as washing, dressing, or providing food and drinks or, on the other, a feeling produced through 'emotional labour' (Hochschild 1983). The two types of care are often conflated yet remain inextricably linked. The term 'emotional labour' was first coined by Arlie Hochschild (1983) who saw that, in addition to physical and mental tasks, flight attendants were also expected to carry out emotional labour in order to reassure passengers in their journey. This theoretical framework has subsequently been applied to many other sectors, including nursing (Ooi and Ek 2010).

Britain has a long tradition of providing tea as part of a healthcare service. A journal dated 1864 demonstrated that tea had already become embedded into hospital provisions of care (Simpson 1864:238–239). Other than milk, tea was the only beverage provided, no coffee or alcoholic beverages; women were permitted four pints of tea and men three. The British public have come to expect 'tea rounds' and 'tea trolleys' as part of healthcare service provided in Britain in both hospitals and hospices. Tea 'trolleys'

---

1 Health Care Assistant, sometimes referred to as 'nursing auxiliary,' perform many of the caring duties such as assisting with washing, dressing, feeding, conducting routine observations, serving meals and, depending on the institution, tea rounds.

are visually present on most wards and are usually purpose-built mobile dispensaries of hot beverages with their own coordinated cyclical routine throughout the day.

In the hospice, offering tea was seen as a good service of care and was a way in which the hospice staff could differentiate their care from hospital care:

> *In the hospice the tea is better . . . it's made in a pot, you are given a mug or a cup with a saucer. You are not given a paper cup with a rationing of milk. There is a communication there, there is a dialogue. It's not just one fits all. It's how do you like it?*
>
> *We have time to make tea, to spend a proper amount of time giving the care you want to give. You get to feel actually happy with the care you've given.*

In keeping with hospice ideology, families are welcomed into the hospice and offered a cup of tea on arrival. The ward clerk told me:

> *The first thing I do when the visitors come is to show them [the] Visitors' Kitchen because, as relatives, you're coming in and you're really distressed and there's a lot going on. The look on their faces when I say: 'You can make yourselves a cup of tea and take five minutes, sit down, you know, your loved one is getting settled into the room'. It's amazing the look on their faces and they go: 'Gosh, great, thank you so much!' . . . 'Wonderful, it's free tea and coffee!'*

The 'visitors' kitchen' was a small little room at the end of a corridor wherein family members could make tea at any time they wished. A kettle sat on the small work surface alongside jars containing tea and coffee provided for by the ward, with decorated mugs housed in a cupboard above. A nurse pointed out that, whilst seen as a welcoming and hospitable gesture on the ward, it also allowed the relatives to be more independent, yet still be involved in supportive care as a family unit. In the hospice, I was told that it was important for the family to feel that they were 'not leading a separate life just because they [were] in the hospice.'

The hospice provision of tea on the wards was also part of a habituated daily routine which included a 'tea trolley,' 'drinks-round,' and newly established 'afternoon tea,' held every day at three o'clock on a table down the corridor whereby a table was set up with a white tablecloth, china cups and saucers, teapot, and freshly baked cakes. Irving (2005:317) has asserted that people's 'perceptions of time and space are generated through [. . .] everyday activities.' However, it has also been asserted that 'illness can disrupt one's ontological perspectives' (ibid:317) and 'the proximity of death slows everything down' (Brian, in Adam 1995). Lawton (2008:57) saw routines in the context of hospice day care are a means of engineering a social construction of time, providing a 'locus of continuity in patients' lives' which would otherwise be characterised by loss and deterioration. Similarly, Hazan

(1980:143) suggested that routines and repetitive activities in an elderly care centre serve to 'freeze' social time for patients and create an 'alternative reality.' It could be said that maintaining social practices helps maintain one's sense of self to prevent a 'social death' (Goffman 1990). A nurse told me:

> *Some people ask for tea out of habit. Even if they don't drink it for like three days, but they'll have it. Because it's part of who they are. They always have their tea at that time. They always have tea with their meal. They always have tea with their sister. That's their habit. It doesn't matter whether they actually get the enjoyment out of the tea itself. Even just the representation of the idea of it is important. It's important to how they act in front of their family. It's important to how they act in front of their friends. 'If I can do this one thing, then I am still OK.'*

Giddens asserted that 'in "doing" everyday life, all human beings "answer" the question of "being"' (1991:48). Furthermore, tea rituals relate to what Giddens calls 'practical consciousness,' being routinised knowledge performed without overt attention. Such performances permit 'ontological security' (ibid:36) through the iterative assertion of normalcy.

This routinised element of 'practical consciousness' in tea making is employed by the Occupational Therapists who use the learnt sequence of tea making as part of a 'functional assessment' of patients. Tea making, I was told, is seen as a 'regular activity' for most patients and a good demonstration of both cognitive and physical ability. There is a habitual, common, but learnt aspect to the practical action of making tea, and this is used as a form of 'reminiscence therapy' for patients living with dementia. Following what the nurse said earlier, being able to make tea speaks to a larger sense of well-being versus decline.

Whilst conducting her ethnographic study in a day hospice, Lawton (2008) encountered patients that wanted above all to 'remain normal for as long as possible.' I similarly observed how the same patients would sit at the afternoon tea table day after day, 'performing' the ritual practice of having tea but often not well enough to fully engage. I was told:

> *I think tea becomes less important to people as they get less well. When they are in bed the whole time and they're given feeding cups with spout on to drink out of or it is thickened with powder . . . the interest in tea disappears. I think it can become less important.*

It appeared that even staff who were not themselves habituated with tea practices could become enculturated to the practices through the construction of a cultural 'right way' to demonstrate hospitality (Rapaille 2006). Billy, who had grown up in the Caribbean, said:

> *It is part of the British culture. So when I came here and I didn't drink tea and I'd go to these people's houses and they'd welcome you . . .*

they'd say, 'would you like a cup of tea? I was never offered anything else but tea. So for people from different cultures, we have come just to adopt tea.

Similarly, Georgette did not drink tea, having grown up in West Africa where it is not the practice to provide tea in care institutions. She developed the practice of offering tea only after she started working in the British hospice:

It's good to do the teas here in the hospice because in this country, some-times it's cold, sometimes it's hot. No matter the weather, everybody likes tea, seems to me. If they are down and you offer them a cup of tea or coffee, drink or chocolate, that lifts their spirit up and lightens their face. Most of the time you get a yes and it calms them down a bit.

Knowing that Georgette did not drink tea, I asked her what she would want to calm her down. She answered, saying, 'If that was me, I'd like a hug.' So, whilst she recognised the cultural practice and had adopted it as a service of care, tea was not meaningful for her personally. Several others, both staff and volunteers, reported accounts where patients or care providers did not drink tea nor share the same meanings associated with tea as emotional care. Schieffelin (1985) in his study of ritual performance in Kaluli séances noted that not all participants will share the same meaning of ritual sym-bols, but that ritual performance socially constructs a situation in which the participants experience symbolic meanings as part of the process. Thus, it follows that the meaning of the ritual is only partly resident in the symbols of which it is constructed.

It also became apparent that the creation of tea as an expected and habit-uated service of care could become problematic for staff providing care, for example, when patients could not or did not wish to drink tea:

Recently we had a patient that didn't like hot drinks. Because you are so used to asking people if they want a cup of tea after a wash or after you have finished seeing them, it was really difficult for me to actually not ask because I knew that she didn't like hot drinks.

Another thing is I think that you really notice how you use giving someone a cup of tea as a way of caring for them when you have a patient who has a PEG[2] or can't take anything orally and then you go to ask them to ask them if they want a cup of tea and then you stop yourself.

Early hospice discourse spoke of the importance of 'emotional involvement' as an 'essential component of hospice care,' which was seen to be a 'complete

---

2 PEG: percutaneous endoscopic gastrostomy. It is feeding tube that is inserted through the nose into the stomach for nutrition or medication for those that are unable to tolerate oral nutrition.

contradiction to the general hospital setting' where healthcare professionals do 'not get involved emotionally with their patients' (Manning 1984:47). Just as 'emotional labour' (Bunting 2016) has been linked to a 'female work ethic' (Smajor 2013), so, too, hospice care itself has been theorised as developing from a 'maternal' (Moller 1996:60) and 'feminine' (Walter 1994:169) ethic in response to 'male technological rationality' (ibid:71). Moral virtues such as a sense of 'caring' and compassion have been socially and historically embedded into nursing practice such that it is an expectation. For doctors who have been described as being 'at a distance from their patients' (Foucault 1993:136), this could be more difficult to achieve. Doctors in the hospice spoke of how they sometimes felt that they needed to 'break down the barriers' in order to demonstrate 'care' for a patient. The practice of sharing a cup of tea had become therapeutically 'emplotted' (Mattingly 1994) into narratives of emotional care in the hospice. Tea was described as 'symbolic' and 'humanising,' it allowed 'objectivising' 'barriers to be broken down.' One of the doctors on the ward gave her thoughts, saying:

> *Sometimes people can feel, I think, like healthcare professionals are not interacting at a purely human level because it's not an equal relationship, no matter how good your communication skills are you can't make the relationship between you and a patient or a patient's relative an equal relationship in the same way you would be equal to somebody you meet at a party and just be socially chit chatting with. It's never going to be that because it is what it is. [. . .] The fact of going off to make the tea and coming back with the tray with the tea and taking the trouble to find out how they like their tea and bringing the milk and the sugar and a couple of biscuits if you can find them. And just that act kind of reminds them that you are another human being and actually you are somebody that, even though this is your job and you're not a loving family member in the same way that they are, that you do care and that you are trying to show compassion.*

Compassion requires a belief or imagination of another's suffering and solidarity through shared experience. Burkitt (2014) in his study comparing emotional labour of nurses in Emergency Department and a hospice saw the importance of controlling affect and emotions. This was predominantly seen not as an individual suppressing their own emotion but as a collective way of dealing with emotions, facilitated by appropriate use of space and the division of labour creating an 'emotional culture' (2014:144) and sharing of affect. It requires both a moral grounding and a conscious judgement as well as skill in language and cultural understanding to be effective (Saunders 2015). Although 'communication skills' are considered attributes that can be taught, it has been debated whether t compassion itself can be taught or if it is simply a 'gift of the Gods' as Socrates has long ago proposed (Pence 1983). The fact that the doctor said that she wanted to 'show' compassion via the tea further demonstrates the material affordance of tea as a warm, filling brew. As something physical, it is more tangible than an emotion, and manifests care in a material form. Furthermore, 'compassion' and 'care giving' have been described as a form of 'gift giving' (Wuthnow 1991:89, Kleinman 2014). Wuthnow (1991:89) explains how the 'gift of care' can be seen as 'a discrete commodity that can have both real and symbolic value' and that the relationship between giver and recipient is characterised by the transfer of a 'gift.' He explains that although service and emotional care are both discrete entities with their own real values, they may also be said to communicate something more amorphous and intangible such as 'good-will,' symbolising one's gestures of compassion or care for another. Thus, one can see how tea comes to be a material form of 'care' and 'compassion.'

The practice of offering cups of tea when breaking bad news or for griev-ing has become culturally accepted in British healthcare. Burkitt studied emotional labour of nurses in hospices and in a busy hospital and found that it was not so much about the individual management of emotion as it was the 'team using a place in which they work to create a situation with its own emotional culture. What is being managed, then, is not an individual emotional system but a situation' (2014:144). The hospice tea ritual can be seen to be the creation of a collective way of dealing with emotional affecta-tion and providing a space to deal with this. Metaphorically, the sharing of a pot of tea can be seen to be the sharing of affect and providing a space for the process of dealing with being emotionally affected by grief or loss. One of the hospice doctors told me:

> There is a value [in tea] particularly in a hospice setting and in situations in particular where somebody is really distressed and they are distressed because a relative is dying or they are dying themselves. These are not things that anyone can fix. There is no fix or solution for the cause of that distress so you just have to find some way of extending comfort to that per-son. It can sometimes be quite a difficult thing to do and it is hard to cap-ture in words what you want to say and the comfort that you want to give.

Palliative care, I was told, is about 'being alongside rather than doing and curing' and that sharing a cup of tea with someone permitted them to 'be alongside.' In a conversation at the hospice I was told:

> I think there is something in our psyche, in our culture that depicts and defines some sense of caring and also flags up the sense of 'I've got a bit of time for you. You know, I'm not going to make you a cup of tea and then let you walk away with it.' There is something about creating a pause and being in the present moment.

There appears to be a creation of a liminal and personal space in time and a focus on the 'present moment.' Bourdieu has postulated that eating with others creates a conviviality that is 'being-in- the-present,' which is thus an 'affirmation of solidarity with others' (1984:183). There is something about this 'being present' that is also reminiscent of Heidegger's concept 'Dassein,' or 'being-there' (1962:27). Heidegger saw 'Being' as a hermeneutic method of thinking and consciousness. In this 'Being-in-the world,' there is an emphasis on the individual, neither as subject nor object but interacting, thinking, and questioning oneself and relation with the world in a present moment. It is thought that Heidegger may have drawn inspiration from Japanese Taoist philosophy and, ironically and indirectly, tea. He received teaching by Kakuzo Okakura and is known to have been given his book *The Book of Tea*. This explores the Zen Buddhist 'Philosophy of Tea,' 'Teaism,' from its roots in Taoist teachings:

> *The art of being in the world [. . .] dealing with the present – ourselves, a moving infinity, [. . .] in a constant readjustment to our surroundings [. . .] to find beauty in our world of woe and worry.*
>
> (Okakura 1906:44)

In the hospice, the occupational therapist, who practised Zen Buddhism, told me about a mindfulness meditation she had started doing with patients using tea as a focus to 'bring the mind to the present moment.' She had been teaching patients and their carers to focus on the tea, concentrating on all aspects of it, the shape of the cup, the physical warmth in the hands, and also creating 'internal warmth' which she described as a 'hug' and comfort as the person drank: 'There are moments in the day when you drink tea and those are the moments that you can look after yourself by being present.' She had found this particularly helpful for the carers who often neglected themselves and their own well-being because of their caring roles. She found that tea was the perfect apparatus for this mindful meditation as it was such an accessible, 'normal,' and 'everyday' thing for most patients.

As Okakura said about the Buddhist tea ceremony:

> *It shows comfort in simplicity rather than in complex and costly; it is moral geometry, in as much as it defines our sense of proportion to the universe. [. . .] a tender attempt to accomplish something possible in this impossible thing we know as life.*
>
> (Okakura 1906:4)

Thinking back to sitting in the hospice clinic as a medical student, I can see how there may have been similar moments of 'bringing back to the present.' There is also research that suggests that in being offered something warm, that one may associate feelings of interpersonal warmth with that person (Williams and Bargh 2008). The physical warmth of tea is often described as a 'comfort,' and it is thought that when offering another a cup of tea, one might associate feelings of interpersonal warmth such as 'kindness' and 'trust.' I was told 'it's a healing warming sensation when someone is in shock,' a 'hug in a mug.' In this sense, as noted earlier, Georgette's preference for a hug speaks to a common desire for warmth as means of comfort.

> *There's something about the drink being hot that makes it quite soothing – that can't be replaced by a cold drink. It doesn't come with that same feeling. When you sit down and have a cup of tea it's 'ahhhh,' it comes with that sense of relaxation.*

For some, the physical properties of tea were important:

> *I am often present when someone has just died. Immediately I think, right, I need to make this person a cup of tea because they will need sugar to help them cope. They need adrenaline to help them cope with this situation, so I will make them a cup of tea to help them through this.*

> *It's not only good emotional well-being, it's good for physical well-being. If you need someone to have a lot of sugar, tea is normally the way we do it.*

> *Tea, here is a form of stimulation, it's a relaxation, it's a calmer. It's a way of relaxation.*

Those with whom I spoke assumed that people would want tea in upsetting circumstances and that the offer of tea was seen to be 'associated with death.' Llewellyn spoke of death as 'a moment in time and a ritualised process' (1991:7). There have always been social rituals around death and dying, particularly to guide people through the grief and mourning processes. It may be that cups of tea have been symbolically inculcated into the modern-day death ritual. In pre-modern times, from the early fifteenth to eighteenth centuries, the 'Ars Morendi' provided both clergy and lay people with a Christian 'script' of what a 'good death' (Aries 1981:29) should involve and 'accepted codes of behaviour' for grieving and dying. This allowed people a 'naive and spontaneous acceptance of destiny and nature' (ibid:29). The secularisation and medicalisation of death has removed such practices from social culture. Whereas prayers may have once been offered to grieving family members, it is now common cultural practice to be offered a cup of tea when someone is bereaved, and it is seen as a socially accepted norm. This culture of tea drinking as a practice for bereavement care is something that has been created, repeated, and reinforced particularly in visual culture. During my research, I found that leaflets and texts on bereavement care often contained pictures of cups of tea or scenes of people sitting around holding cups of tea yet made no reference to the practice in the body of the texts. Hallam and Hockey (1967) have explored the Western historical cultural production of material culture of death and memory. Throughout history, material objects that are significantly important during death rituals often have connotations of transience to reflect the dying or decaying body, yet have the permanence of memory. There is an impermanence of a cup of tea in that it is consumable, but also that the warmth of the drink will begin to dissipate much like the body of the deceased.

Whilst offering people a cup of tea was seen as a vehicle for providing emotional care and facilitating conversation if one is alongside, I also discovered it was used in the context of avoiding difficult or emotionally burdensome situations. I was told it was 'a good prop,' 'almost when you don't know what else to do' but also as a way of ending a difficult conversation. I was told by a nurse:

> *I remembered when I first qualified and it was down to me to be there when bad news was broken and things like that. If I was really struggling . . . 'Oh my god, I'll make a cup of tea'. It was almost like 'oh what do I do now, oh yeah, I'll make a cup of tea.'*

In her ethnographic work on the English, Kate Fox has asserted that 'putting on the kettle' and 'making a cup of tea' is 'the perfect displacement activity' (2005:312). Similarly, I was told that both the 'tea bar' and the visitors kitchen could be a means of physically leaving one's relative to enact one's emotions away from the bedside.

As a practice, offering tea is embedded and encouraged in hospice institutional care. In the hospice I was told that when someone died, 'it's normally when the posh crockery comes out, for some reason.' Having a predicted or prescribed practice, however, may also become problematic and conflict with hospice ideologies of 'person-centred care' approach of the hospice if routinised. I was told that in another hospice, a particular 'tea set' was brought out when bad news was broken. The patients and relatives became aware that this particular tea set signified that bad news was on its way and it became known as the 'death set' and so people would anticipate the conversation. This was not a practice that the hospice wanted to portray and so the said tea set was made redundant.

The fieldwork demonstrated the complexity of care in the hospice. Tea was very present in the hospice and became intertwined with practices of care, as a service of care and in emotional care. Social practices of tea have been created such that tea has now become a cultural artefact in patient care and bereavement rituals.

Hospice care has largely developed out of an anti-institutional model seeking to provide a homelike environment for patients and their families. Incorporating habitual routines with tea to some extent replicates the image of home for some and maintains a sense of normality and self at a time of decline and loss. There has also developed a sense of enculturation such that it is seen as a social norm to offer tea in certain situations as is seen by people who have come to adopt the practice when working in the hospice.

The physical warmth of tea allows it to stand in place for human warmth, nurturance, and vitality at a time of great vulnerability and distress for patients and their families. Tea was also used as a cultural and ritual symbol, as a tangible representation of emotional care and compassion. In offering tea, a liminal space is created in which conversations can be facilitated and emotions enacted. Sharing this liminal space allowed healthcare professionals to 'be alongside' and demonstrate their humanity, which was seen as important in showing compassion. Tea has, consequently, become a key material of care in this British hospice. The two kinds of care, both as practical service and as emotional labour, become entwined and conflated in tea, separate yet inextricably linked.

References

Adam, B. (1995). *Timewatch: The Social Analysis of Time*. Cambridge: Polity Press.

Ariès, P. (1981). *The Hour of Our Death*. Trans. Random House. New York.

Bourdieu, P. (1984). *Distinction*. Cambridge, MA: Harvard University Press.

Bunting, M. (2016). Who cares: The emotional labour of an undervalued, underpaid workforce. *The Guardian* 15 March. Accessed www.theguardian.com/society/2016/mar/15/care-workers-undervalued- underpaid-radio-3]

Burkitt, I. (2014). *Emotions and Social Relations*. London: Sage.

Clemens, K.E., B. Jaspers and E. Klaschik (2003). The History of Hospice. In D. Walsh (Ed.), *Palliative Medicine*. Philadelphia: Saunders Elsevier.

DuBois, P. (1980). *The Hospice Way of Death*. New York: Human Sciences Press.

Einöther, S.J. and V. E. Martens (2013). Acute effects of tea consumption on attention and mood. *The American Journal of Clinical Nutrition* 98(6):1700S–1708S.

Farrell, Mary (2002). *From Cha to Tea: A Study of the Influence of Tea Drinking on British Culture*. Republished from 1660. Castelló de la Plana: Publications de la University Jaune.

Foucault, M. (1993). *The Birth of the Clinic*. London: Routledge.

Fox, K. (2005). *Watching the English: The Hidden Rules of English Behaviour*. London: Hodder.

Giddens, A. (1991). *Modernity and Self Identity: Self Society in the Late Modern Age*. Oxford: Polity Press.

Goffman, E. (1990 [1959]). *The Presentation of Self in Everyday Life*. London: Penguin.

Golby, J. (2015). Tea is a national disgrace. *The Guardian* 27 May 2015. Accessed 25 June 2018. www.theguardian.com/commentisfree/2015/may/27/tea-national-disgrace-beverage-british.

Hallam, E. and J. Hockey (1967). *Death, Memory and Material Culture*. London. Bloomsbury.

Hazan, H. (1980). *The Limbo People: A Study of the Constitution of Time Universe Among the Aged*. London: Routledge & Kegan Paul.

Heidegger, M. (1962). *Being and Time*. Trans. J. Macquarrie and E. Robinson London: S.C.M Press.

Hochschild, A.R. (1983). *The Managed Heart: Commercialisation of the Human Feeling*. Berkeley: University of California Press.

Illich, I. (1976). *Limits to Medicine: Medical Nemesis: The Expropriation of Health*. London: Marion Boyars.

Irving, A. (2005). Life Made Strange: An Essay on the Re-inhabitation of Bodies and Landscapes. In W. James and D. Mills (Eds.), *The Qualities of Time: Anthropological Approaches*. Oxford: Berg, 317–329.

Kleinman, A. (2014). How we endure. *The Lancet* 383(9912):119–120.

Lawton, J. (2008). *The Dying Process. Patients' Experiences of Palliative Care*. London: Routledge.

Llewellyn, N. (1991). *The Art of Death: Visual Culture in the English Death Ritual c1500–c1800*. London: Reaktion Books.

Manning, M. (1984). *The Hospice Alternative: Living with Dying*. London: Souvenir Press.

Martin, E. (2014). The 'H' Word. *eHospice*. Accessed 28 August 2016. www.ehospice.com/uk/Default/tabid/10697/ArticleId/11189/

Mattingly, C. (1994). The concept of therapeutic 'Emplotment'. *Social Science & Medicine* 38(6):811–822.

Moller, D. (1996). *Confronting Death: Values, Institutions and Human Morality*. Oxford: Oxford University Press.

Munley, A. (1983). *The Hospice Alternative*. New York: Basic Books.

O'Brien, T. (1993). Pain. In C. Saunders and N. Sykes (Eds.), *Terminal Malignant Disease*. London: Hodder & Stoughton.

Okakura, K. (1906). *The Book of Tea*. London and New York: G.P Putnam's Sons.

Ooi, C.S. and Ek, R. (2010). Culture, work and emotion. *Culture Unbound: Journal of Current Cultural Research* 2:303–10.

Orwell, G. (1946 [1970]). *The Collected Essays, Journalism and Letters of George Orwell (Vol. 4)*. In S. Orwell and I. Angus (Eds). London: Penguin.

Pence, G. E. (1983). Can compassion be taught? *Journal of Medical Ethics* 9:189–191.

Quinlan, P., J. Lane and L. Aspinall (1997). Effects of hot tea, coffee and water ingestion on physiological responses and mood: The role of caffeine, water and beverage type. *Psychopharmacology* 134(2):164–73.

Quinlan, P., J. Lane, K. Moore, J. Aspen, J. Rycroft and D. O'Brien (2000). The acute physiological and mood effects of tea and coffee: The role of caffeine level. *Pharmacology Biochemistry and Behavior* 66(1):19–28.

Rapaille, C. (2006). *The Culture Code: An Ingenious Way to Understand Why People around the World Buy and Live the Way they Do*. New York: Broadway Books.

Saunders, C. (1965). Watch with me. *Nursing Times* November 1965.

Saunders, J. (2015). Compassion. *Clinical Medicine* 15(2):121–124

Schieffelin, E.L. (1985). Performance and the cultural construction of reality. *American Ethnologist* 12(4):707–724.

Sharangi, A.B. (2009). Medicinal and therapeutic potentialities of tea (Camellia sinensis L.): A review. *Food Research International* 42(2009):529–535.

Simpson, J.Y. (1864). *The Medical Times and Gazette: A Journal of Medical Science, Literature, Criticism and News*. London: John Churchill & Sons, 238–239.

Smajor, A. (2013). Reification and compassion in medicine: A tale of two systems. *Clinical Ethics* 8(4):111–118.

Twycross, R. (1992). *The Dying Patient*. London: Christian Medical Fellowship.

Walter, T. (1994). *The Revival of Death*. London: Routledge.

Williams, L.E. and J.A. Bargh (2008). Experiencing physical warmth promotes interpersonal warmth. *Science* 322(5901):606–607.

Wuthnow, R. (1991). *Acts of Compassion: Caring for Others and Helping Ourselves*. New Jersey: Princeton University Press.

Verma, H. (2013). Coffee and tea: Socio-cultural meaning, context and branding. *Asia – Pacific Journal of Management Research and Innovation* 9(2):157–170.

8 'Regenerative medicine event'

Cells, soybeans, and a repurposing of ritual in Japan

Jesse Bia

Setsubun with Etsuko

Etsuko was 79 years old, a lifelong Tokyoite, and not one for frivolous conversation. She was stern and solemn, but surprisingly sociable nonetheless. Fiercely independent, living on her own as a widow in a luxury downtown apartment complex suited her fine. Her financial and familial circumstances were comfortable. She had several successful grown children, and though she lived frugally, she was affluent. Her fiscal means allowed her to maintain a noteworthy degree of autonomy, which she valued enormously.

Etsuko's current situation was a stark contrast to her childhood. As a young girl, her father was shipped out to fight in the Pacific and never returned. She survived the American firebombings of Tokyo that destroyed her home, killing her mother and sister. She spent her formative years being raised by her maternal grandparents on the outskirts of the city. Etsuko's grandparents steeped her in the local folk traditions, practices, and remedies of the Kantō plain. It was applied knowledge she carried into her octogenarian years.

Etsuko's single overriding obsession was her own health. She referred to 'kenkō' ('health/well-being') constantly in conversation.[1] Every time I conducted research with Etsuko we engaged in a health-related activity: workshops, medicinal gardening, kampo classes on traditional Japanese herbal medicine and philosophy, guided hikes for exercise, even a beauty expo – she went for the skin care products. Etsuko was the co-organizer of an elderly social club for Tokyoites over-65 who attended multiple activities a week, and many of these events were health-oriented. I originally met Etsuko during one such activity: a kampo class she attended with the club, taught by another participant I was working with at the time. Even proceedings that were not overtly about health, such as local *matsuri* ('festivals'), acquired a *kenkō* aspect due to the values Etsuko and others attached to them, as is the focus of this chapter.

---

1 All translations of dialogues and source material from Japanese are the author's.

In early 2015, I received a typically succinct email from Etsuko stating that I would be accompanying her social club to a 'regenerative medicine event' ('*saisei iryō gyōji*'). We would rendezvous at Shōsōji, a prominent Buddhist temple in Tokyo.[2] The temple was centrally located, so I assumed we would walk from there to the 'regenerative medicine event.' However, on arrival that day, I realised the 'regenerative medicine event' was apparently the traditional Setsubun festival taking place at the temple. I was perplexed.

I was in the middle of two consecutive years of on-site participant observation fieldwork examining perceptions of regenerative medicine ('*saisei iryō*') in Japan, namely the manifestations and reasons – the 'How?' and 'Why?' – of its current widespread public acceptance (Bia 2018). In short, regenerative medicine is the collection and processing of biomaterials from human bodies and the subsequent transplantation or injection of these biomaterials into patients, with the aim of partially or completely curing damaged or dysfunctional organs, tissues, and cells. This is predominantly accomplished using stem cells, both native and induced, via cellular therapies. Often these cells will be manipulated *in vitro*, bioengineered to propagate around an inductive scaffold/extracellular matrix and/or induced into a pluripotent state.[3] The resultant stem cell/bioengineered tissue(s) generated will then be (re)inserted into the body. Once inside, the cells collectively act as a catalyst: multiplying and influencing the body to heal itself around the insertion *in vivo*.

Saisei iryō is well-known and popular throughout Japan. Therefore, it may be initially surprising to note that most treatments are either still in clinical trials or laboratory testing, not in translatable use with patients yet. However, this current absence of translatable treatments allows regenerative medicine to manifest as a series of 'imaginaries,' where a lack of direct implementation begets a conceptual space wherein individuals ascribe and project their own idealised meanings, forms, and anticipated uses onto *saisei iryō*.[4] The present malleability of a *saisei iryō* definition greatly contributes to its personal and societal acceptance in Japan: *saisei iryō* can still be whatever individuals want it to be.

Even with definitional flexibility considered, a 'regenerative medicine event' at a temple was unusual, and a first for my research at the time. The majority of my fieldwork up to that point took place in hospitals, clinics, laboratories, and homes of the infirm, much less so Buddhist temples and

2 The names of all participants and specific locations in this chapter are pseudonyms.
3 '*In vitro*' refers to processes occurring outside of a living organism, such as in a test tube or petri dish, whereas '*in vivo*' describes processes which occur within the body of a living organism.
4 I utilise 'imaginaries' here as 'imagined forms of social life and social order reflected in the design and fulfilment of scientific and/or technological projects' (Jasanoff and Kim 2009:120; also see Jasanoff 2015).

Shinto shrines. In terms of biological influence, contemporary Buddhism in Japan is largely utilised for practical rites and issues surrounding death (Long 2005; Stone and Walter 2008; Kawano 2010). But it is not often used for health maintenance, and rarer still the application of tangible medicine beyond the selling of *omamori* amulets to ward off various maladies. I was not sure how Setsubun at a temple could acquire a medical component, let alone relate to regenerative medicine.

I met Etsuko and 15 members of the social club at Shōsōji's main gate. I recognised a few members from introductory kampo class where I first met Etsuko, which took place at a kampo school where I was both conducting research and training to become a certified kampo pharmacist *(kampoyakushi)*. I promptly learned we were staying at Shōsōji for Setsubun. We had arrived an hour before the official start, but the temple grounds were already a hive of activity. A large makeshift four-track elevated runway had been constructed in front of the stairs to the *hondo* (main hall). As a group, we moved to the back left, and were soon consigned there by barrier ropes and bodies. The group was eager to stay close to the runway, lightly jockeying for the best positions.

Setsubun is a Japanese folk celebration dating back centuries. It marks the end of winter and the beginning of the New Year cycle according to the traditional lunar calendar, usually February 3rd or 4th. The most prominent ritual of Setsubun is *'mamemaki'*: the scattering of roasted soybeans – *'fukumame'* ('fortune/luck beans') – which ward off evil spirits/demons to increase luck and fortune in the coming year. Originating as secular regional folk custom, Setsubun today is celebrated at both temples and shrines across Japan. As a secularised practice, there are also municipal events at city halls. While not a national holiday, many individuals of all ages will attend in the morning or on lunch breaks. It is a common primary school field trip. In a pinch, one can buy any number of mass-produced *fukumame* in a convenience store on the way home from work.

When the festivities officially started at Shōsōji, approximately 2,000 people surrounded the runways. The crowd was diverse: middle-aged, late teens, families with children. But elderly men and women were the very clear majority. Our section up front appeared almost entirely elderly.

The pre-*mamemaki* procession began, starting at the main gate and cutting through the entire temple complex before going up the back entrance to the *hondo*. It was led by Buddhist priests in full regalia, methodically banging staffs on the ground and holding incense. They were followed by a group of *gagaku* musicians. The musicians were followed by roughly one hundred children and their teachers from a local primary school, each pupil wearing mock temple robes and homemade green headbands; they would be casting out *'oni'* ('demons' – represented here by adults in costume) later on. They were followed by a few hundred laypeople in temple jackets born in the various Years of the Ram/Sheep (ranging from 1919 to 2003), which

2015 was, meaning some of these individuals were 96 years old. They were responsible for throwing soybeans into the crowd during *mamemaki*.

Ten minutes later, *mamemaki* began. More accurately: *mamemaki erupted*. As Year of the Ram throwers took up position along the runway railings, the crowd surged forward. Hand-wrapped packets of roasted soybeans were tossed into the sky. Instantly, I was in the middle of an elderly mosh pit – a fierce one too. It was public behaviour I had not witnessed in Japan before, including the subway: pushing, shoving, and diving onto asphalt. One older man wiped out hard in front of me and was quickly helped up, only to dive down again a second later to grab a packet. The social club had dispersed: it was each person for oneself. The tossing continued; priests and apprentices continuously refilled boxes with *fukumame* packets from supplies in the *hondo*. Emcees instructed the crowd over loudspeaker to shout '*Soto!*' ('Outside!') and '*Uchi!*' ('Inside!'): an abbreviation of the traditional Setsubun chant of '*Oni wa soto! Fuku wa uchi!*' ('Demons out! Luck inside!'). A group of men in the middle of the runway nexus methodically pounded out *mochi* rice cakes with huge wooden mallets in time with the chanting, a staple practice of many public Japanese ritual celebrations. *Mamemaki* appeared an exercise in orchestrated chaos.

After ten minutes of throwing, there was a respite. The primary school children then rushed onto the runways, chasing away costumed demons by throwing their own *fukumame*. I used the time to retreat further and catch my breath, where I found the majority of the social club perched in a row on a ledge. They all appeared unscathed by the melee. Most were eating their *fukumame*.

'Where are your fukumame?' Etsuko asked.

'I didn't catch any.'

'That's no good. You need to go back.' The initial throwing was only the first of many rounds throughout the morning and afternoon.

'Leave your backpack here. Go.'

I attended Setsubun at Shōsōji the following year as well, again with Etsuko's social club, in addition to a *mamemaki* in a rural Kanagawa Prefecture town. I went to Shōsōji alone over the two days prior to view Setsubun preparations and converse with laypeople volunteers – many of them elderly themselves – putting the whole event together in conjunction with temple officials. After speaking at length with the social club, elderly volunteers, and additional elderly participants over the two-year course of my fieldwork, it became clear that the meaning and purpose Setsubun was changing for them. It was not about luck and fortune anymore: it was about maintaining health in the face of longevity. Under this rubric, in both form and function, Setsubun linked with *saisei iryō*. As will be explained in this chapter, this was indeed a 'regenerative medicine event.'

From 'luck' to 'health'

As children and teenagers in the immediate post-war years, many members of Etsuko's social club had thrown *fukumame* in the yard and street to cast away *oni* and bring luck in the upcoming year. Most ate the *fukumame* too. Only one individual had never participated in Setsubun until joining the social club. But now, no one in the group scattered soybeans that were gathered during *mamemaki* outside homes or businesses anymore, though some did use commercially bought soybeans for this purpose. Now, for elderly participants, *fukumame* gathered during Setsubun's *mamemaki* ritual were solely for eating.

Even amongst those who grew up eating the *fukumame*, the consumption ritual had changed. *Fukumame* were not merely eaten: one had to consume the exact number of soybeans that corresponded to age, plus one. 'A healthy year ahead, that's why the one extra *fukumame*,' Etsuko explained. This was a recent development for those in the social club.

The roasted soybeans being thrown from the runway came in hand-sealed packets, assembled at and by Shōsōji. Braving the storm, I was able to grab one of these packets each year. There were enough beans in each to just cover my age, plus one. But many of the elderly in the social club needed three packets of *fukumame* to reach their age, plus one. Supplies were limited and *mamemaki* – at least the initial rounds – had become a contact sport (another new development for those in the club). General consensus amongst the club was that skipping Setsubun was OK, but beginning *fukumame* collection without finishing was ill-advised: it would actively contribute to poor health. Not bad 'luck' *(fuku)*, but bad 'health' *(kenkō)*. 'We all must finish, that's why I sent you back,' explained Etsuko, as the club nodded in agreement. Starting the *mamemaki* process and not finishing was analogous to beginning a course of antibiotic treatment and stopping halfway through: ineffectual and potentially hazardous to health.

I inquired multiple times about the commercial *fukumame* one could purchase: why not buy a bag at 7-11 and eat the corresponding number? 'They're not effective,' exclaimed one club member. 'I throw those outside my home,' extolled another, and the club approved. 'These are Shōsōji's *fukumame*. They can influence health. Store-bought *fukumame* can't do this.' Again, a chorus of approval. The source of the *fukumame*, at least for personal healthcare, was critical.

The parallels to medical prescription are evident: medicine (soybeans) issued from a medical authority (Shōsōji) has increased potency, and definitely more potency than over-the-counter medicine (soybeans from convenience stores). During Setsubun, medical authority was temporarily projected onto the temple.

I inquired about the intense jostling for *fukumame* packets – was it not dangerous? While some self-consciously admitted it might be, Etsuko stood firm: 'It's what needs to be done. Health requires great effort. You have to devote time. . . . We're here early every year.' The ritual rush for limited *fukumame* packets had taken on a new meaning for these elderly: health maintenance and illness prevention. As articulated by Etsuko's social club: yes, one could go to the store and buy mass-produced *fukumame*, but the potency to influence health would be absent. Expanding on this correlation, it is the difference between quickly purchasing over-the-counter medicine or visiting a medical authority for specialised, targeted, more potent medicine via prescription. The latter is a product that cannot be obtained without investing time, effort, and approval from an authority. The investment and approval are vital to the expected outcome.

To extrapolate a repurposed meaning of Setsubun to all elderly Japanese would be a wildly inaccurate generalisation. But this specific example *is* representative of a wider pattern of medicalising rituals amongst the elderly population in the wake of the demographic shift, which becomes all the more clear when comparing how younger generations experience the same rituals differently from their elders.[5]

This repurposing of Setsubun is *not* universal: it is specific to the elderly. Each time I attended Shōsōji's Setsubun, I remained long after the social club left. The attendee demographic changed significantly over the course of the day, as did the material properties of the *fukumame*. There were differences from earlier in the morning. The number of attendees increased, reaching a peak of about 4,000 by 1:00 p.m. The attendees were no longer predominantly elderly; they went from the majority to a small minority. From midday on, attendees were now men and women in business attire on lunch breaks, usually in groups, along with uniformed high school students. Families with small children increased. Behaviour changed too: the mad dash was gone. Despite the increase in numbers, there was a marked decrease in physicality. No less enthusiasm, but no more desperation for *fukumame*: fun, not friction. No one was diving on the ground anymore.

The material properties of the *fukumame* thrown changed too: the hand-wrapped packets of roasted soybeans specific to Shōsōji were phased out. By midday, bags of commercially available *fukumame* were being tossed – the exact same bags one could purchase around the corner in 7–11. During the initial *mamemaki* tossing in the morning, a few of these commercial bags were thrown alongside Shōsōji's hand-wrapped soybeans: the commercial bags were left untouched on the ground while elderly pushed for the packets. Later in the day, when a commercial bag was grabbed, individuals would open it and casually eat the roasted soybeans by the handful, paying no obvious attention to the number consumed. Many more commercial bags

---

5 Setsubun was not the only traditional ritual where I witnessed and documented a newly infused medicalisation over the past five years amongst elderly participants: *tondo-yaki*, *shichifukujin meguri*, and *Kōshin-kō* practice all had novel medical aspects. Though not included here, they will be the subject of planned future analyses.

were tossed later than packets earlier: families and groups of friends could load up on multiple bags with enough to augment lunch and maybe scatter at home, the office, or school. Setsubun was still about luck for non-elderly generations. But as vocalised by elderly participants, for them, *fukumame* were now objects for health. Which leads to the question: what factor(s) instigated this change of meaning amongst this specific demographic section of the population?

A burden in the 'super-aged society'

The answer to this question is that Setsubun at Shōsōji is taking on a new dimension for Japanese elderly in the wake of Japan's demographic shift.[6] The *mamemaki* ritual, until recently, was mainly concerned with the warding off of *oni* to bring luck. For most Japanese, it still is. But for the elderly I directly worked with, and the many more I observed, the focus had changed from luck to health, for reasons largely tied to intense national demographic pressures and their impacts on healthcare.

Japan is a rapidly ageing country. The ageing is so intense that a neologism was created to describe the phenomenon: '*chōkōreika shakai*' ('Super-Aged Society'). In a population of 126.8 million people, 33 million (26%) are over the age of 65: more than one in four Japanese.[7] Comparatively, in 1990, right before the catastrophic collapse of Japan's bubble economy *(babaru keiki)*, the over-65 population stood at 14.9 million and 12% of the population: a 16% increase of 18.1 million individuals over 65 years old to the present. The most commonly cited statistic(s) tied to Japan's population is life expectancy: Japan has the highest average life expectancy in the world at 85 years old (81 for males, 88 for females), and the highest median age at 47 years old. An ageing population does not inherently imply disaster, so long as said demographic can be supported. At present, Japan's healthcare infrastructure is being stridently tested, because the ageing population is compounded by additional straining demographic trends.

The most significant of these coinciding trends is that Japan's overall population is also shrinking. The 2015 Japanese census marked the first time the total population literally shrank, declining 0.7% from 128.1 million in 2010 to 127.1 million in the five years between national censuses: a drop of 947,000 people. The result was expected. Still, crossing the threshold from 'reduced growth' to 'active decline' sent a collective shock through the

6 The 'demographic shift' is my own term. I use this construction for both relevance and applicability. It is a purposely broad term that covers larger Japanese demographic trends and statistics, but also myriad changing social patterns that underlie said statistics, specific to Japan, that fall outside the normal purview of macro-demographic analysis.

7 Unless otherwise noted, all demographic data in this chapter are official government statistics from the Japan Statistical Yearbook of the Ministry of Internal Affairs and Communications 2017 (Sōmu-shō 2017).

Japanese press, politics, academia, and citizenry alike during my fieldwork: negative potentiality actualized, accompanied by morose – occasionally frantic – responses and realisations. Demographic prognosis is dire: official government estimates place the 2025 Japanese population at 120.6 million, a decline of almost 6.5 million from the present, with the total number of over-65 population rising to 36.6 million, a rise of 4%. By 2040, the total population is projected at 107.2 million, with the over-65 population rising to 38.7 million, a full 36% of the overall total. Japan's population is ageing and shrinking at distressing rates. The resultant rising percentage of elderly to total population puts a tremendous strain on public healthcare infrastructure and familial networks of care (see Matsumoto 2011; Wu 2004; Traphagan 2000, 2003, 2006).

This demographic shift is felt strongest amongst the elderly, particularly infirm elderly, and those caring for them. Elderly are living longer and there are fewer individuals to help take care of them, in both professional and familial capacities. In Japan, with demand so high, spaces in care homes are largely reserved for elderly with critical medical needs (see Koyama 2016). As such, many infirm elderly do live with family; over 3.8 million elderly Japanese receive supplemented in-home care by medical professionals while living with family members (Rōkenkyoku 2016:13). The demands of home care can breed resentment and depression amongst caregivers, giving rise to another neologism: 'kaigo tsukare' ('caregiver exhaustion'). Many households are not eligible for all of the benefits of kaigo hoken ('Long-Term Care Insurance'), implemented in 2000 and meant to alleviate the burdens of home care, due to its reliance on outdated and inaccurate models of family structure. Nonetheless, the responsibility to provide familial care for elderly family members – possibly at the cost of employment or having children – is acutely felt by younger generations. Many non-elderly participants I worked with were experiencing this strain first-hand.

Many elderly I worked with were worried about becoming a care burden on their families, when their own health problems could potentially interfere with the finances and personal lives of familial caregivers. It was a concern voiced equally by both healthy and infirm elderly throughout my fieldwork: a potent anticipated fear, regardless of individuals' situational and medical realities. Increasingly, elderly in Japan are searching for self-initiated, preventative, proactive health management options so as to avoid burdening others: the minimisation of social and familial disruption through biological intervention. Etsuko valued her autonomy for its ability to keep her from becoming a self-perceived burden as much as the daily practical benefits it afforded.

Regenerative medicine is seen by many in Japan as a multivalent antidote for the medical maladies of the growing elderly population. Research and laboratories are championed and often financially supplemented by the federal government. Whether in its pure biomedical form, or as a series of projected imaginaries (or both), many Japanese regardless of age are encouraged by the new medical prospects.

The highest profile translatable regenerative medicine in Japan is for the treatment of chronic degenerative diseases that frequently affect the elderly: cardiovascular and respiratory disease, diabetes, and neurodegenerative conditions. Cellular therapies are also being developed and implemented for chronic disabilities common to the elderly, including sensory impairments and osteoarthritis. Currently, the most nationally celebrated regenerative medicine work in Japan is a clinical trial to treat wet-type age-related macular degeneration with induced pluripotent stem cells, a condition which affects upward of 700,000 elderly Japanese.[8]

Regenerative medicine is viewed as an answer to a set of contemporary healthcare problems exacerbated by the demographic shift. In treating degenerative health conditions that affect the elderly demographic, there is also the potential to ameliorate the family strains resultant from elderly care. The early days of translatable treatments mean that individuals still have a profound ability to personalise what *saisei iryō* actually *is*, ranging from wider macro social implications to the micro properties of materials involved. This conceptual flexibility is the most dominant theme I continue to document with participants. Elderly are living longer, with fewer health-care resources and social safety nets than before. Maintaining health – main-taining *autonomy* – in the face of this longevity is highly desired. Setsubun has naturally acquired an additional contemporary purpose: medical treat-ment. The material products of Setsubun became medicine.

Present circumstances went so far as to shape memories: when I initially asked Etsuko why she scattered *fukumame* outside her grandparents' home as a teenager, she said 'To prevent illness *(byōki)*.' She corrected herself – it was 'to bring luck in the upcoming year' – but the verbal slip was revealing as to the new meaning of Setsubun to her and her cohort.

'Repetitive self-treatment'

Setsubun has become medical for many elderly in the wake of the demo-graphic shift. But how does it fit under the rubric of 'regenerative medicine'?

There is a telling linguistic linkage and logographic similarity at work here. Because written kanji in Japanese have multiple signifiers, the con-struction of Japanese neologisms is incredibly important, as said construc-tions demonstrate deliberate intent to represent a specific meaning.[9]

'Saisei iryō' – 'regenerative medicine' – is one such neologism. Written as '再生医療,' it is created from two pre-existing words: '*saisei*' (regen-eration) and '*iryō*' (medical treatment/care). The kanji representing '*sai-*,' '再,' which constitutes the first logogram in '*saisei*,' is principally used as an

8 Wet-type age-related macular denegation is a chronic degenerative disease in which abnor-mal blood vessels form underneath the macula of the retina causing a gradual deterioration of vision.
9 Zhu (2013) has conducted similar medical anthropology work with written logograms in the context of Chinese linguistics.

attached prefix to denote repetition over time. The second kanji of 'saisei,' '生,' is meant in this context as 'life,' but also with strong connotations to the self ('I/myself/me'). 'Iryō,' '医療,' is medical treatment, particularly treatment sanctioned – though not necessarily administered – by an official healthcare authority. Thus, while not conceptually taken as the following, the strict literal logographic depiction of the kanji for *saisei iryō* is 'repetitive self-treatment.'

Saisei iryō is a neologism, and there are obvious differences between the literal logographic representation and what people interpret as the concept represented. But while individuals say and read '*saisei iryō*'/regenerative medicine, a basic deconstruction of the terms illustrates that there are elements of *repetition*, *the self*, and *proactivity* underscoring the term. Etsuko's association of regenerative medicine with a repeated self-initiated health intervention facilitated through an (albeit temporary) medical authority – in this case Setsubun at Shōsōji – is entirely understandable. Setsubun now exemplified those exact characteristics. For Etsuko and cohort, Setsubun has become a verbatim enactment of *saisei iryō* as it is written.

The practice of *fukumame* ingestion further engenders linkage to treatment procedure via a large number of cellular therapies. A biological entity(s) is induced and/or provided by a medical authority. A very small amount is taken into the human body with minimal invasiveness. Biological and social disruption are both marginal. The biological entity then acts as a catalyst for self-treatment, influencing the body to repair/maintain itself. The body is not *healed*: the body *heals itself*. The locus and orientation of healing is internal and reflexive.

Amongst the elderly Japanese I worked with, Setsubun had become a repurposed folk ritual where material properties of *fukumame* are reconceptualised to have a new medical function. These properties mirror the form, functions, and purpose of stem cells and cellular therapy: regenerative medicine. There are strong parallels in perception and practice, and the influence of the demographic shift – particularly how it impacts the elderly – is paramount to each.

Accompanying the logographic link between *fukumame* ingestion and regenerative medicine is also a categorical one between the soybean and tangible medicine(s), built on the realities of modern medical practice and treatment in Japan. Engendering a connection between the soybean and effective, potent, prescribed medicine is not an abstraction here. In both industry and academia, the frequent inaccurate separation of botanicals and biomedicines is often made by those with vested interests in doing so. When one considers the prevalent use of kampo amongst the Japanese population – through the exact same healthcare rubrics, legislations, and professionals as biomedicine – this categorical association becomes visible. Due to the status and use of botanicals as effective prescribed medicine via kampo, *fukumame* as potent medicine is not a categorical realignment.

I have documented the extensive integration of kampo and biomedicine in Japan through participant narratives and socio-historical analysis elsewhere

(Bia 2018). However, it is worth briefly delving into select connections here, in order to illustrate how botanicals are afforded the same functional status as biomedicines in Japanese healthcare, issued by the same medical authorities, for the same medical purposes. Kampo, too, is part of the wider movement amongst Japan's elderly for proactive personal healthcare management; again, as mentioned previously, I first met Etsuko in a public kampo class to which she had brought her social club for that exact reason.

Kampo medicines are composed of herbs, autonomous and/or combined, used in a variety of physical forms. Kampo prescription is a common feature of medical practice in Japan. Since 1967, the Ministry of Health, Labor, and Welfare (MHLW) has included coverage of approved kampo medicines under *kokumin kenkō hoken* (National Health Insurance), currently numbering 148 formulations, and allows prescription of additional kampo medicine that does not fall under said coverage as well. Presently, 90% of Japanese biomedical physicians ('*isha*') will prescribe kampo medicines to patients as part of regular practice (Yoshino et al. 2016:118). Kampo pharmacies and practitioners will make referrals to biomedical clinics and hospitals, and vice versa. Many kampo pharmacists also have degrees in biomedical pharmacy as well: during my time spent researching and training in a kampo pharmacy and school, over 95% of my fellow aspiring *kampoyakushi* had already earned a collegiate pharmacy degree. Though the diagnostic methods and physiological conceptions of kampo practice and biomedicine are distinct, both are used as complementary parts of an integrated Japanese healthcare structure. They operate in tandem: parts of the same unified system, with overlapping governing legislations, professionals, and patients.

Kampo medicines themselves are subject to approval by authorities, identical to biomedicines, even when not covered by *kokumin kenkō hoken* or prescribed by *isha*.[10] The raw ingredients come from a preapproved list of 165 botanicals defined in the official *Nihon yakkyokuhō* (Japanese Pharmacopoeia) issued by the MHLW. Kampo medicines and ingredients must meet strict evidence-based standards approvals. No kampo product can be prescribed or sold without passing official MHLW efficacy tests. Approval is granted solely on evidence-based criteria, measured within the same quantifiable framework used for biomedicines. Kampo must meet the same relative efficacy standards as biomedicine for authorisation. This produces a healthscape where categorical medical materiality is defined less by material properties than by the ability to meet a standard criterion of proof and subsequent approval by authorities.

Kampo – botanicals – are experienced by patients through the same ritual of prescription as biomedicines: a ritual conducted by the same physicians

---

10 Kampo medicines not insured under *kokumin kenkō hoken* are mainly in-house formulations of individual kampo clinics and pharmacies. Though not under coverage, they must still meet the same evidential criteria as prescription kampo/biomedicine and be authorised by the MHLW.

and sanctioned by the same authorities. Repurposing *fukumame* is a small categorical variation: a process of simply shifting the soybean under the wider shared umbrella of medical botanicals and biomedicines that already exists in Japan.

Silver technology

For many elderly, both the stem cells of regenerative medicine and (increasingly) the *fukumame* of Setsubun are representative of what Susan O. Long (2012) has called 'silver technology' in Japan. The word '*shirubā*' (the Japanese rendering of 'silver') is used throughout Japan in conjunction with products and services specifically meant for the elderly. '*Shirubā shīto*' ('silver seats') are reserved seats for elderly on trains and buses; '*shirubā hōkōki*' ('silver cars') are devices used to facilitate transport for elderly with limited mobility; '*shirubā jinzai*' ('silver resource centres') help a growing number of unemployed elderly find jobs. *Shirubā* designates materiality specific to function within the elderly population.

Long's initial formulation of 'silver technology' refers exclusively to assistive medical devices: wheelchairs, hearing aids, hospital beds, and more. However, this definition can easily be expanded to include biologics without theoretical conflict, which is what I propose here. Not only is such an expansion reflective of biological realities on the ground (including Japanese healthcare legislation), but also the semantics of the term itself: '*shirubā*' featured heavily in the public discourse of '*shin gijutsu*' ('new technology') in the '*kenkō būmu*' ('health boom'), in coverage of both regenerative medicine and elderly care. This includes medical procedures, pharmaceuticals, and biologics, along with aforementioned assistive medical devices.

Elderly in Japan are 'consumers not only of devices [silver technology], but of the meanings they carry' (Long 2012:120). With both *fukumame* and stem cells, the overall and overlapping meaning is one of health maintenance. There is also the desire for autonomy and independence, as is vividly demonstrated by Etsuko herself: not wanting to become another care-dependent statistic of the demographic shift and an encumbrance on family members. They represent proactive personal management of – and novel options for – healthcare: semiotic exemplars of control. Therefore, the unproblematic redefinition of objects *(fukumame)* alongside the acceptance and incorporation of the new (stem cells) features heavily as part of the larger *shirubā* healthcare narrative in Japan. Both are equally emblematic of how Japanese elderly are reformatting and utilising materials to make sense of the new medical realities of the demographic shift.

Soybeans as/with stem cells

Etsuko introduced the initial Setsubun outing as a 'regenerative medicine event.' No doubt this is partially because she knew I was actively researching regenerative medicine. But she would not have articulated it as such if she did not also see the validity in doing so.

In Etsuko's case, the connection between regenerative medicine and consuming *fukumame* at Setsubun was conscious. Like with *in vivo* regenerative medicine, small, biological entities were introduced into the body in non-invasive ways. Said entities were approved and issued by a medical authority, even if only temporarily, as in the case of Shōsōji. The perceived form and function of *fukumame* and stem cells is comparable here: the *fukumame* function like stem cells. They do not 'cure' or 'treat' directly, but galvanise and instigate the body to heal and treat itself. The logographic representation of '*saisei iryō*' reinforces this connection: keeping with the literal written depiction of '*saisei iryō*,' Setsubun *fukumame* ingestion is also repeated, reflexive, and sanctioned by a medical authority. Categorically, viewing botanicals as potent medicine via kampo, alongside biomedicines, is common in Japanese healthcare: *fukumame* are merely being shifted under this integrated medical rubric.

Stem cells are not soybeans, nor are soybeans stem cells. But though the strict biological form may differ, under these conditions the function now overlaps. The *fukumame* were adopted into a health/cellular/regenerative treatment rubric(s) by participants. *Fukumame* provide means to potentially avoid becoming a burden on one's family. Stem cells, via cellular therapies of regenerative medicine, have the potential to remedy health conditions of elderly who already feel they are a burden. Both are empowering, and the goals of health maintenance and avoidance of inconveniencing family are mutually shared.

This continuity runs deep. Here, Japanese ritual(s) now shares corresponding uses with *saisei iryō*: unification of function and (re)purpose between traditional practices and future technologies. Not only are Japanese individuals engaging with regenerative medicine through medical treatment and popular culture, but they are also doing so through repurposed constructs which have been drawn under the conceptual canopy of *saisei iryō*, imbued with medical aspects they did not previously have. In the case of Setsubun, the initial repurposing concerns the functional material properties of the *fukumame* gathered during *mamemaki*, which are analogous to stem cells and biomedical treatment, respectively. Again, by consuming *fukumame* in this manner and for this purpose, Etsuko and her cohort are performing the verbatim enactment – the living embodiment – of *saisei iryō* as it written.

The material properties of *fukumame* and stem cells are not identical. However, in Japan, their use and function are beginning to intersect: the intended purpose and medical impact on/within the material body is remarkably similar. *Fukumame* are now silver technology, and for growing numbers of elderly Japanese, Setsubun is a repurposed ritual.

As the demographic shift escalates strains on both national health infrastructure and familial care, elderly Japanese are searching for their own self-initiated forms of practical health management. Increasingly, they are turning to themselves – internally – for health maintenance. This prompted the proactive repurposing of Setsubun for 'health' outcomes. Setsubun is now less about '*Fuku wa uchi!*' ('Luck inside!'), and more concerned with personal healthcare: health inside. 'Luck' is no longer sufficient; it lacks the specificity and efficacy participants are seeking. For elderly Japanese, these new personal *in vivo* applications leave much less to chance.

References

Bia, J. (2018). Sunshine technology and dream biology: Perceptions of regenerative medicine in Japan. PhD. University College London.

Jasanoff, S. (2015). Future Imperfect: Science, Technology, and the Imaginations of Modernity. In S. Jasanoff and S. Kim (Eds.), *Sociotechnical Imaginaries and the Fabrication of Power*. Chicago: University of Chicago Press, 1–33.

Jasanoff, S. and S. Kim (2009). Containing the atom: Sociotechnical imaginaries and nuclear power in the United States and South Korea. *Minerva* 47:119–146.

Kawano, S. (2010). *Nature's Embrace: Japan's Aging Urbanites and New Death Rites*. Honolulu: University of Hawaii Press.

Koyama, Y. (2016). Oya no kaigoe no kikon josei no kakawari to sedaikan no ryōteki kankei [Quantitative analysis of parental care involvement by married women]. *Jinko Mondai Kenkyu* 72(1):28–43.

Long, S.O. (2005). *Final Days: Japanese Culture and Choice at the End of Life*. Honolulu: University of Hawaii Press.

Long, S.O. (2012). Bodies, technologies, and aging in Japan: Thinking about old people and their silver products. *Journal of Cross-Cultural Gerontology* 27:119–137.

Matsumoto, Y. (2011). *Faces of Aging: The Lived Experience of the Elderly in Japan*. Palo Alto: Stanford University Press.

Rōkenkyoku [Health and Welfare Bureau for the Elderly – MHLW]. (2016). *Long-Term Care Insurance System of Japan*. Tokyo: Nippon-koku Seifu.

Sōmu-shō [Ministry of Internal Affairs and Communications: Statistics Bureau]. (2017). *Japan Annual Statistical Yearbook 2017*. Tokyo: Nippon-koku Seifu.

Stone, J. and M. Walter (2008). *Death and the Afterlife in Japanese Buddhism*. Honolulu: University of Hawaii Press.

Traphagan, J. (2000). *Taming Oblivion: Aging Bodies and Fear of Senility in Japan*. Albany: State University of New York Press.

Traphagan, J. (2003). Contesting Coresidence: Women, In-Laws, and Health Care in Rural Japan. In J. Traphagan and J. Knight (Eds.), *Demographic Change and the Family in Japan's Aging Society*. Albany: State University of New York Press, 203–228.

Traphagan, J. (2006). Being a Good Rōjin: Senility, Power, and Self-Actualization in Japan. In A. Leibing and L. Cohen (Eds.), *Thinking about Dementia: Culture, Loss, and the Anthropology of Senility*. New Brunswick: Rutgers University Press.

Wu, Y. (2004). *Care of the Elderly in Japan*. London: Routledge.

Yoshino T., K. Katayama, Y. Horiba, K. Munakata, R. Yamaguchi, S. Imoto, S. Miyano, H. Mima, and K. Watanabe (2016). Predicting Japanese Kampo formulas by analyzing database medical records: A preliminary observation study. *BMC Medical Informatics and Decision Making* 16(1):118–136.

Zhu, J. (2013). Projecting potentiality understanding maternal serum screening in contemporary China. *Current Anthropology* 54(S7):S36–S44.

9 The form that flattens

Kelly Fagan Robinson

Introduction

In this chapter, I explore negation of DEAF[1] authority due to transformational movement between material forms, what Bechter (2009) defines as a *conversion* from five-dimensional modes of expression to a negatively transduced text existing in two dimensions. I focus here on a form called 'How Your Disability Affects You,' a crucial proof-collection step in the UK's Personal Independence Payment (PIP) claiming process. I argue that the divergent modalities and affordances present in the process of attempting to contain the ineffable stuff that the 'Affects You' form seeks to capture, in fact, may hide embedded epistemic differences between the deaf sign-language-using claimants and the institutions that might support them. So it is that the textual materials generated by this process are dangerously oversimplified and are more representative of the PIP's mandated process of re-presentation than they are of the PIP claimant herself.

Field background and context

An estimated 2,255,500 deaf and 'disabled' people in the UK applied for Personal Independence Payment (PIP) between 2013 and 2016.[2] The Equality Act 2010 defines 'disability' as:

---

1 Within scholarship centring on deaf people, 'deaf' mainly refers to 'not-hearing' (conditionally); and 'Deaf' mainly refers to 'not-Hearing' (culturally). These are thus largely delimited by their opposite, hearing-centred concepts. 'Deafhood' (Ladd 2003) is used to name the negotiation across such cultural/conditional boundaries, seen as a process of continually becoming *'dDeaf'*. In contrast to these terms, 'DEAFness' (Gulliver 2009) is construed neither as a foil to hearing, nor to connote the negotiation as one navigates across boundaries of becoming. Rather, it is centred on DEAF-specific authorship and is thus a lens onto the structures underlying the broader emic concept of DEAF World and the mapping of DEAF people's lived experiences.
2 Unless otherwise noted, all PIP data are sourced from relevant UK governmental reports, up to date at time of writing.

(a) a physical or mental impairment [that]
(b) has a substantial and *long-term adverse effect* on [the person's] ability to carry out normal day-to-day activities [emphasis mine] (Equality Act 2010)

Linking disability to its '*long-term adverse effect*' creates the imperative of proving that such effects exist. Claiming for benefits based on 'disability effects' thus requires a peculiar kind of evidence collection. Explaining, encapsulating, and evaluating each person's *affective* experiences – 'affective' here defined as both the externalised as well as somatic effects brought on by disability – is a nuanced and complex process. In particular, when conducting the PIP assessments, claimants are typically reliant upon describing, proving and, ultimately, placing a numeric value on what constitutes 'substantial and long-term adverse effect.'

During doctoral research (2013–2017) into myriad modes of deaf people's communicative performances, resources, and authorship, I[3] volunteered at a deaf-led advisory centre that specialised in supporting deaf clients access to frontline public services. From 2013, the Department for Work and Pensions (DWP) began to move from administering a benefit called Disability Living Allowance (DLA) to the new PIP scheme. As was highlighted in February 2018 by the 'PIP and ESA [Employment Support Allowance] Assessments: Claimant Experiences' report to the House of Commons Work and Pensions Committee (hereafter referred to as the PIP/ESA Report),

> assessment processes function satisfactorily for the majority of claimants, but they are failing a substantial minority [. . . Claimant testimonies were] striking and unprecedented [numbering nearly 3500 individual testimonies].
>
> (2018:19)[4]

According to the PIP/ESA Report, one in 20 PIP and ESA claims received benefits only after challenging and overturning the DWP's initial decision. Of the 290,000 people for whom this was the case, 227,000 were claims related to PIP. During the roll-out of PIP (2013–2017), disabled claimants, many of whom had been supported by DLA previously, were called upon by the DWP to process a new claim. This included many deaf beneficiaries.

Challenges due to shifts in assessment protocols ensued, difficulties that could in the first instance be attributable in some part to key differences between the two benefits. First, DLA is a benefit that provides financial support towards needs that are the result of disability or illness, designed

3 I am a hearing person with UK NVQ Level 6 BSL qualification/competency.
4 The report, dated 17 January 2018, was published on the UK Parliament website on 14 February 2018.

to alleviate any additional financial burden resulting from such conditions. DLA has, therefore, always been determined on a non-means-tested basis and was payable

> regardless of employment status [. . .] based on proxies – care and mobility – as research at the time of DLA's introduction showed that they were the greatest sources of extra costs.
>
> (DWP 2013:2)

DLA is still administered for children up to 16 years and maintained for people over 64 years. By contrast, PIP evidence collection is subtly but importantly different in that it is meted out on the basis of perceived *long-term adverse effect* brought on by disability. As the advice on the 'How Your Disability Affects You' form stipulates:

> We don't need to see general information about your condition – we need to know how you are personally affected.
>
> (DWP 2015:3)

This raises a second significant challenge in the new PIP criteria: at several key stages of the process, claimants are asked to provide testimonies or artefacts that attest to the fact that such adverse effects have both been experienced and witnessed by the claimant and/or by those around them. These proofs are not based only on diagnoses or material evidence, but rather on negative *qualia*, here meaning the 'sensory experiences of abstract qualities such as heat, texture, colour, sound, stink, hardness, and so on – [as they] focus attention on prototypically "material" entities' (Chumley 2017). Here, qualia looks to the materialisations of *adverse effect* as these are connected with disabling conditions on/in/through a person's body.

For example, when conducting the PIP evaluations, assessments are typically reliant upon describing, proving, and ultimately placing a numeric value on what constitutes 'substantial' long-term adverse effect; a high enough overall score will result in a successful claim. However, there is a requirement embedded in the claiming process of proof, specifically how one's disability (whether physical, intellectual, or psychological) demonstrably exhibits ongoing hardship. This first requires the claimant's self-understanding to be framed as not only 'disabled' but also 'impaired.' Additionally, despite the fact that most effects of disability begin somatically – and thus can be experienced only by the claimant alone – current methods of proving need for PIP require external corroboration in order to quantify such qualia. Invariably, the needs and understandings of the claimants and the mediators of the claimants' 'effect' are, therefore, held in tension. Each participant – the claimant, corroborating witnesses, form-fillers, and evaluators – brings unique feelings (or perceptions about other people's feelings) to that process. The result can be confusion for the participants, but even more problematically, it can mean an unwitting erasure of the key claimant details on the paper form, as I will now describe. This calls into question whose effects (or *affects*) are quantified in the evaluation. It further begs the question: which message is being received and assessed, and which communicative form will convey this most accurately?

Bodily form at odds with institutional form: 'How Your Disability Affects You'

PIP benefit was, for most clients at the advisory centre where I volunteered, an essential source of income. For Tuck,[5] a profoundly Deaf, sign-language-using client at the centre, PIP was a critical component in her attempts to reconstruct her life post-hospitalisation for paranoid schizophrenia. But her claiming process was far from the straightforward five steps depicted in www.legislation.gov.uk/ukpga/2010/15/pdfs/ukpgaen_20100015_en.pdf DWP literature's 'PIP claimant journey' (2014:1) as follows:

1 Thinking about claiming
2 Making a claim
3 Telling your story (told by the in-filled form 'How your disability affects you')
4 Assessment
5 Decision

In 2016, Tuck was in her mid-40s. She'd had a diagnosis of paranoid schizophrenic for more than two decades. Tuck's initial application for DLA was centred on her deafness and was filed by her parents during her infancy, and as far as she understood, she had been granted the benefit on an indefinite basis. The idea that this vital benefit *might* be something to 'think about claiming' did not fit with Tuck's experiences. It was simply something that had always been there. 'Thinking about claiming' was an aftershock that occurred only once Tuck had received a letter informing her that she must file a claim for PIP because her unthought-of DLA was ending. Receiving this letter led to stress and emotional upheaval, leaving Tuck *upset and confused . . . why are they taking DLA away from me?* The letter itself was, therefore, a key source of her disabilities' adverse effect. The PIP system rendered her vulnerable to the removal of her income (on which she relied in order to pay rent) by virtue of her effects of disability having to be proven, thereby forcing her to question both her body and her stability, contorting both to fit.

Tuck came into the advisory centre because she needed to initiate the new PIP claim by phone.[6] Like many other deaf people, when she needs to make a phone call she must seek intermediary support. Roughly four out of every five appointments at the deaf advisory centre where I volunteered

---

5 Anonymised.
6 At the time of writing, a videophonic BSL interpretation option was also being offered, but this was not yet available at the time of Tuck's initial application.

are made in order to gain telephone access to various services. For Tuck and other clients, there were consequently many other steps between receiving the letter concerning DLA conversion to PIP, 'Thinking about Claiming,' and then 'Making a Claim.' Tuck visited the centre five or six times throughout the claiming process to phone the DWP and their partners and to gain assistance with various forms. In each meeting, I used my voice to represent Tuck's interests over the phone in my capacity as volunteer advisor. I did not represent my voice *as* Tuck's voice like a BSL interpreter would, but rather explained to the call-handler at the DWP that Tuck and I were sat opposite one another, working through the process and forms together, signing back and forth with me offering voice-over.

Our first meeting's priority was to request the re-initiation of her expired option to claim, though the reader should note that this ultimately represented an even greater imperative: the need to reinstate her income in order to prevent Tuck becoming homeless. So far, we were united in our cause. However, as I engaged in a charged manner with the DWP call-handler, Tuck reclined in her chair, covering her eyes, withdrawing; thus, the witness-able effects brought on by her emotional experiences at that moment were noticeably different from my own. Importantly, during the phone call, it was my role to convey the urgency of Tuck's situation rather than her demeanour at that point in time. Tuck's seeming lack of engagement was at this early stage already partially obscured from the claim because of the aim of our call. The process from the first call, therefore, became clouded by competing affects: Tuck's present-time actions of seeming disinterest in that moment of calling, the urgency I perceived she felt given how upset she was about the need to claim, and my expressive capacity as vocal-prosthetic, representing what I perceived to be her underlying intent. I raise this because it exemplifies that though I acted as her bridge to the encounter with the DWP and it to her, I also in part occluded it. This is a trend that occurs throughout all claims processes: when an intermediary is involved, the claimant message will always be influenced by that intermediary. Filtration of the call through another person instigates a partial or total dispersal of the visible effects of claimant's disabilities in any given moment.

Once Tuck received the 'How Your Disability Affects You' form, she returned to fill this in with me. In addition to the first six pages asking for basic address details, birthdate, lists of conditions, illnesses, and disabilities, as well as the evidence to back up such diagnoses, there are a further 29 pages designed to illustrate these effects. The PIP demands of the claimant an explicit picture-painting of life impediments brought on by her disability. Tuck has two conditions that she self-classifies as 'disabilities' – her deafness and her paranoid schizophrenia (although she has additional illnesses as well she did not want to discuss). For each of the named conditions, she would have to explain her daily challenges, pain, and instances of incapability in order to qualify for PIP.

The format of the form appears to be seductively easy. The claimant and advocate can simply tick one of three boxes in each section: 'YES,' 'NO,' or

'SOMETIMES.' But beneath each set of tick boxes sits a box about the size of a drink coaster offering the possibility (though not the requirement) of further explanation of how each answer of 'YES,' 'NO,' or 'SOMETIMES' impacts upon the individual's life, particularly if in negative ways. Though these boxes are not demanded, in my experience, they must be filled in if claimants want to give their distant and anonymous PIP assessor a better idea of what the benefit will mean in their lives and why it is necessary. This imperative was both somewhat hidden (included only as 'extra') and also at odds with Tuck's view of herself as someone getting better. In her desire to appear 'fine,' Tuck initially remained reserved about the history of her paranoid schizophrenia: she did not want to discuss it because she was *well now*.' It was, therefore, challenging for me to ascertain the details behind her claim. She spent the first and second, two-hour advisory appointments insisting that she was *fine*; she needed no support; she was improving; she was *better*. Proving impairment sat at odds with her aimed-for clinical progression from illness to wellness.

Thankfully, Tuck came back to the centre repeatedly. While she insisted that she was *fine* during the early appointments, this noticeably shifted in the third. Only then, after many more 'fines' had been signed, did I ask if she still wanted to claim. She nodded, '*yes*.'

ME: *I think we need to revisit the purpose of this form. This is different from DLA, you know?*
TUCK: *How different?*
ME: *Even though this form asks you to tell the DWP how you are now, we also need to tell them how you have been, and what kinds of things need to be in place in order for things to continue to improve in the future.*
[Tuck shook her head 'NO.']

At length, Tuck sighed, looked at me and then watched her right hand as she raised it and made it flat, palm facing downward. As she told me the following, her right hand maintained what I came to realise represented her bodily/conditional timeline. She extended her right hand, beginning just above her right shoulder, pointing outward, palm flat to the ground. As she explained, the hand followed the invisible variegated terrain ahead. Tuck's eyes followed that timeline as it peaked and troughed. I present here, in textual form, my understanding of her signing – a representation once removed. Because of this removal, I represent her words not CAPTIALISED – as they would be in conventional British Sign Language (BSL) notation – despite the fact that she used BSL signs (if not always BSL grammar) throughout our appointments. This, the reader should note, is the way I wrote out what she performed for me upon the 'Affects You' form:

I was at college when I was diagnosed as paranoid schizophrenic . . . attending college for a degree in IT. I was highly social – lots of diverse

groups of friends, hearing, deaf, church friends, uni friends – I was
highly productive – but always up and down.

As she described this, her face conveyed the moments of palpable happiness
(peaks) during which point her planed hand would shoot skywards. Her
face followed the hand, her mouth opened, her upper back arched slightly.
These upward swings were followed by troughs, a bodily composed crush-
ing sadness. During the dips of her right hand, the intensity of her expression would change accordingly; when her right hand peaked, her shoulders
and torso would extend upward to show joy, when it troughed, Tuck would
shrink into herself, eyes downcast, shoulders hunched as if each spinal bone
segment curled inward, checking with a sideways glance on her extending planed right hand. Tuck was drawing time and feelings with her body,
projecting towards me (by default, a representative of her future) from the
shoulder anchor of her static but un-dateable past-tense, mirroring the
dynamism of the timeline depicted by the right hand. At times, she looked
somewhat frenzied, at others, seeming almost asleep. When I asked again,
when were you first diagnosed? she continued, having reached its highest
point, her right hand began to plummet steadily, gathering speed as it went.
As it plummeted, she signed with her left hand to clarify:

In 1999. . . it was 1999, yes, and suddenly, one day as I was walking
to class
[Her happy face looked around at all her unseen friends, greeting
them as they passed by, waving with her left hand, nodding, smiling.
Then her expression clouded, and she squinted her eyes, flinching.]
I couldn't tell which people were my friends and which were my hal-
lucinations. The light was dancing in funny ways. I stopped going out
in daylight because the sunshine skewed my vision
[At this point, her right hand completed the plummet, reached the
furthest point possible on her leg, and her entire body exhibited an
attitude of having crumpled after a horrible (physical) crash, curled-in
at odd angles in her chair.]

Tuck explained that in earlier years, when a crash occurred, her father
would manage her finances – pay her rent, her utilities, her tax, manage her
bank account, and so on – while her doctors and nurses as well as a host
of social workers would manage her food intake, water, medication, physical activity, and anything else that could contribute to her mental stability
improving. However, by the time I met her, she did not seem to have her
parents involved in her life, though she did not offer the reasons why. These
episodes continued to occur from 1999 through the following decade and a
half, always with a similar pattern.

This last time, back in August [2016], that was because of the medica-
tion. They had me on the wrong medication and they brought me back

to the hospital to fix it. Because it wasn't me, it was the medication. But
1999 . . .
    [Here her right hand retracted, as if it was a rewinding film, and dove backward in time-space, following in reverse the peaks and troughs she had conveyed to this point, landing at the lowest trough.]
    . . . that was me,
    [She frowned at her fallen palm and paused.]
    but this time . . .
    [Her right palm rapidly re-traced the same pathway she has just unwound, now fast forwarding to the recent past, an 'after' in relation to 1999 but a 'before' in respect to today, depicting the line in the same fine detail, face and body following her hand with their corresponding happiness-highs, and desperation-lows.]
    . . . was the medication . . .

As she finished explaining her history from 1999 through to the present, her right hand landed right near my left shoulder as we sat, face-to-face. She looked at the hand and then at me, and signed:

And now, now my medication is better. And now, you see, I'm really better. Always a bit better. I'm fine. Understand?

What I understood was that 'fine' represented for Tuck both the hopeful expression of how she wished to be seen 'now,' but was also the expression of her aspiration for the future. I hesitated because I was wondering how I could re-convey the world that she had just shared from my haphazard and scattered notes? How to reconcile the complex but cohesive and contained performance I had just witnessed, with the requirement of the form to trans-duce that specific production, flattening it into the mono-linear, sequential PIP form? I was conscious that if Tuck continued to insist she was 'fine now' this could potentially undermine her PIP claim. Yet it was imperative that I represent on the paper exactly what she was telling me. She did not appear aware of the paradox this generated.

    Though Tuck might wish to project fine, she had also clearly articulated in her performance that she was continuing to have to actively manage the various effects of her conditions. It later emerged that by the time she was hospitalised in 1999, she had already deteriorated and had had previous medical interventions; these were undated – lost in Tuck-time. At her worst moments, she would not leave her bed; she stopped eating because it was too frightening to go out for food. Sometimes, when it was very dark out-side, the sunlight-induced hallucinations would fade, and she would feel better. But during the daytime, the phantoms rose with the sun and she would hide. I stared, stuck on the first page, and the columns that needed filling in. They read:

'Health condition or disability' and 'Approximate start date'.

The 'effects of disability' that Tuck had just performed simply did not match what the 'Affects You' form was asking her to tell.

After taking the claimant's name and basic details, the form [Figure 9.1] asks only:

Q2   About your health conditions or disabilities [. . .]

(i)   use page 6 of the information booklet

Q2a   Please use the space below to tell us:

a   what are your health conditions or disabilities
b   approximately when each of these started?

This part of the form is one half of an A4 page. The allocated box for explanation of the 'conditions' or 'disabilities' is 12 lines and has divided the 'conditions' from their placements in time via separation into the two columns on the form. The column on the right is there to record the date of when each pathology first occurred. Once that date is written, the condition becomes punctuated in time and has a past, 'before' the illness. It also has an implicit continuing-present in which the named pathologies are still relevant; otherwise, they would not be includable in the present tense conditions dictated by the form. The form also gives clear instructions to separate these pathological conditions and the moments in which these occurred (these are in-filled on the first page) from their effects by issuing the guidance at the bottom of the note: *If you need more space or want to tell us anything else, please continue at Q15*, Q15 features near the very end of the 39-page form. As I attempted to fill in the form, I became conscious that on the basis of these instructions, information concerning the effects of her conditions, despite being wholly connected to diagnosis because they represented the symptoms which signalled her pathologies, were not yet includable or even allowable at this stage in the evidence collection.

Tuck's telling was also, crucially, representative of her DEAFness as she expressed it using BSL. It included known signed grammatical features like multiplicity of spaces, and simultaneity of events/feelings/places. Her use of BSL and gesture exhibited the effects of her deafness through the five dimensions of sign language she mobilised: by communicating within 'the geometry of the field in which the constituents of a message are displayed,' Tuck made use of 'three dimensions of space and one of time' (Stokoe 1980:368) and constantly employed 'intensity' (Labov 1984; cf. Bechter 2009), a communicatively enacted affective fifth dimension exhibited through facial expressions, shifting body positions, and movement dynamics. These components allowed Tuck to not only remember what had occurred, but also to 'climb' (Gulliver 2009) back into her experiences of deafness and disability to display their effects. Climbs can be seen as one form of DEAF narrative

Section 2 - About your health condition or disability

ⓘ Use **page 7** of the **Information Booklet** to help you answer these questions.

Q2a - Tell us in the space below:

- **what your health conditions or disabilities are, and**
- **approximately when each of these started.**

Health condition or disability	**Approximate start date**
Example: Diabetes	May 2010

We will ask you how your health conditions or disabilities affect how you carry out day-to-day activities in the rest of the form.

If you need to add more please continue at **Q15 Additional information**.

PIP2 October 2016

4 of 33

Figure 9.1 Page 4, question 2a of the 'How Your Disability Affects You' form.

called *visual vernacular* (VV), 'a technique that makes a visually told story more dynamic through change of perspective [similar] to what occurs in a movie with change of camera angle' (Siple 1994:349). Employing VV, Tuck became the places, spaces, creatures, weather, and people from her lived experiences of disability. Through use of these DEAF modes of authorship, Tuck directly conveyed the effects of and on her deaf body. She, therefore, also made explicit the role of DEAFness within her own life by using DEAF modes of expression.

Making use of such 5D communicative resources allowed Tuck to further demonstrate the impacts of psychosis on her life, allowing her to both re-turn into, and also comment as a witness on her own paranoid schizophrenic episodes. Though there may have been a technical diagnosis date – *it was 1999, yes* – Tuck offered a contextualising, bodily grounded scenario: she parsed each moment of her disabilities, making them 'now' all over again. The repetition of each performance placed the beginning of her disabilities as indefinite – constantly re-starting as she re-presented them. The issue became how to capture these dynamic moments of performance in order to make them includable in the form. It seemed impossible to 'capture' and map Tuck on paper, with all the moments of her conditions/illnesses and their supposed causes; everything came in what to me felt like a random order and did not fit in a linear, left-to-right timeline.

As if reading my mind, Tuck released her bodily timeline. It looked as though she unravelled the picture she had created with her body – releasing the extended timeline arm, face losing all expression – returning to totally neutral. Before she had been 'painting in the air' (Gulliver 2009) in front of me, re-turning five-dimensionally within those moments. Now, she sat all the way back in her chair and her illuminated face shadowed. She held up her hand to say *hang on . . .* and pulled over a stray scrap of turquoise paper and a black pen. On the paper, she drew the same timeline (Figure 9.2), with such exacting precision that I could tell she had done this many times before. The dynamism of her performance just one moment earlier receded entirely, and she was once again inert – numbed, as if her face mirrored the same flattening required by the form.

Tuck slowly pushed the paper forward. The timeline drawn on the paper mirrored the one she had created with her body. Each peak – the same as those she portrayed by her right hand moving through time, and her body and expression arching and swooping between euphoria and devastation – was now written down alongside a date positioned adjacent to the drawn line. It was readable, punctuated, dated, but it contained no sense of her feelings because her intensity dimension had been eliminated. It was the intensity of her grammar that had most clearly revealed to me how these moments *continued to affect* her. Now every moment was marked down on the line and dated but flattened for me and for the PIP form; the affective dimension was absent.

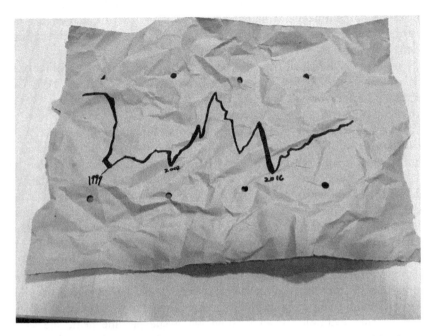

Figure 9.2 A timeline topography of Tuck's illness trajectory, mapped by her to illustrate her gestures.

Source: Image copyright of Kelly Robinson.

Disparate times call for disparate communicative support

Because time and again Tuck's affects were not in-line with the questions that the form was asking, her 5D performances highlighted a clear disparity between two distinct *chronotopes* or 'timespaces' (Blommaert 2015:106): (1) her own re-turning time within events and their effects in the now-as-always and (2) the chronological historical time of the 'How Your Disability Affects You' form. But even as Tuck attempted to body forth the evidence of negative effect required by the 'Affects You' form, her performed proof was matter out of place because in the document the form parses the condition/start-date (sought in Q2) from the proof of impact (included much later in Q15). To include the information where it should 'naturally' belong (according to Tuck's performed DEAF chronotope) thereby works against Tuck because the inclusion of this data earlier in the form is in direct contravention of the instructions given. The instructions in the initial part of the form are also at odds with the general guidance offered in the 'Claimant Journey' information disseminated by the Department for Work and Pensions (DWP 2015:3): *We don't need to see general information about your condition – we need to know how you are personally affected.* Tuck's chronotope, the time-space that she re-presents in order to include it in her testimony, is, therefore, at odds with the sequential and linear chronotope of the paper form.

The disparity between these two chronotopes also affects the quality of the evidence itself. Tuck re-presents her lived experiences *as* her key mode of proof – in other words, her DEAF authority born of her deaf body serves to articulate both the ongoing 'when' of Tuck's deafness as well as its 'how' as it affects her repeatedly over the ever-extending long term.

Additionally, by exhibiting her communicative resources and requirements using a performed, transient, but ever-enactable form, Tuck also proved the ongoing communication support she would continue to require in the face of English-based institutional processes. For example, when these meetings occurred, she could not fill in the form herself because, although she read everything, she frequently required explanation of anything I wrote on her behalf, and she would forget what we had already discussed, requiring a further review of the written material. When she tried to read the form herself, she found the questions very confusing and also struggled to hold a writing implement for more than a few seconds because her hands shook from her medication. She would visibly panic if she attempted to write without success.

In another example, when I asked when she became deaf, she asked me to phone her uncle to discover the answer. She was surprised when he explained that she had been born deaf rather than becoming deaf later. She did not believe this was true. This phone call became a critical proof of one key ongoing long-term adverse effect: *suspicion*. She indicated that she was just as suspicious about the beginning of her deafness as she was of her initial diagnosis of paranoid schizophrenia – *suspicious and upset*. Weeks after this call, Tuck would periodically stop our form-filling sessions to ask: *do you believe I was born deaf?* She several times suddenly shifted into another scene concerning a woman who had not given her the right change at a convenience store. Tuck suspected it was because the woman knew she was deaf and was cheating her. Problematically, in the 2D form, this connection between her 'start-date' and such long-term 'effect' was all but invisible, included only as supplementary asides in a separate section of the form.

Relatedly, the shop-lady's suspicious manner also made Tuck reticent to return to that shop despite it being the only one open at night. She often went without food when she was unwell (which led to extensive weight loss). And though the 'Affects You' form does specifically ask about the ability to cook fresh food, when I asked about this, Tuck responded, '*Of course! I'm perfectly capable of cooking a meal!*' However, it was clear this was not the entire story.

The form's question reads:

> Please tell us about your ability to prepare a simple one course meal for one *from fresh ingredients*. This includes things like:

- food preparation such as peeling, chopping or opening a can, and
- *safely* cooking or heating food on a cooker hob or in a microwave oven.

We want to know if you can do this safely, to an acceptable standard, as often as you need to and in a reasonable time.

(DWP 2015:6 emphasis added)

While Tuck might have had the capacity to cook, she had already admitted that she would at times be unable to leave her flat for food because she was too unwell (and afraid) to do so. Though she had begun eating again by the time we filled in the 'Affects You' form, after talking things through multiple times, it turned out that she had stopped eating only a few months earlier, immediately preceding her most recent hospitalisation. Her ability to acquire fresh food was impacted by her suspicions about the shop-woman by whom Tuck believed she had been cheated. Tuck's ability to maintain a fridge full of 'fresh' food was, therefore, contingent on her ability to successfully procure food outside her home. She frequently went without food, would lose body fat, and then her medication dosages would likely need adjustment, without which she would drastically increase her risk of a breakdown.

Again, this is information that does not really sit within the question asked but is relevant to the broader question of how disability affects Tuck as an individual, and how she as an individual is able to *safely* feed herself. This past-time emotional state of 'being/feeling afraid' is, therefore, relevant to the present-time question of '*safely* preparing food' through the body it continues to affect. The form's completion requires only that boxes must be ticked, responding 'YES,' 'NO,' or 'SOMETIMES.' After questioning colleagues, I found that most form-fillers would simply tick the boxes that signalled the client did not need help in order to cook. A form-filler's mediations are thus directly responsible for communicating (or not) the deeper and ongoing effects of the disability. Too often the claimant's flattened-to-paper-form lacks the depth of description exhibiting *how* she gets to be fine and is unwittingly flattened further. The DEAF individual contends with how to fit her unique experiences of body and society within the rigid confines of PIP paper format, in a way that can still suitably and recognisably exhibit long-term adverse effect.

Despite this gap in communication, Tuck still identified that the disparity between DEAF communication and 2D texts could be used to guide the way she conveyed her effects of *wellness*. She explained many times that she could not have been born deaf because, as she told me, '*I think in English*.' This phrase '*I think in English*' thereafter emerged as a key point of differentiation in Tuck's attempts to convey order to those around her. Tuck explained to me that her paranoid schizophrenic condition meant that her clinicians and social workers were continuously checking to see how 'ordered' her mind was. This alongside the role that formal English played in her assessments (most of her support network were hearing, English speakers and writers), meant she had come to see English language as the primary mode by which she could convey *I am fine*. I did periodically notice that though she would mainly use BSL for the friendly chit-chat at the start of our meetings, she would then shift to sign in English grammar rather than in BSL grammar. I had thought she did this to ensure that I could understand because I am a non-native signer. Tuck explained that this was only part of the reason: she intentionally used English grammar to convey what she perceived would be considered to be internal order and sound mind.

Tuck explained that she had gotten into this communication habit with her teachers at university, who would communicate most effectively by writing assignments down. Communicative disconnects occurred constantly in Tuck's life, not only with her teachers but with hearing friends and later her support networks due to mismatched bodily, socio-historic, temporal, spatial/geographical contexts in which the act of understanding each person's language is embedded. The 'cognitive leaps' (Wilson and Sperber 2012) that happen when two communicative partners have enough elements in common to fill-in-the-blanks might not occur if the communication gaps are too wide. Recognising this, Tuck claimed she later returned to using English grammar-patterns in meetings with her doctors, to prove how *'well and in-control'* she was. She believed that rather than using the less receivable DEAF-shaped multidimensional re-turns in time-space, it was easier to use more recognised English particularly in the flat paper-based PIP communications.

Kidd and Carel have written about the ways that in the healthcare domain the lack of common ground between teller and listener has a profound impact on interactions between patients and their clinicians, because

> breakdowns in the epistemic relationship can result in ill persons having negative subjective experiences of healthcare, such that they might come to associate hospitals not only with sickness and suffering, but also with confusion and isolation.

> (2014:173)

This insight seems particularly relevant to PIP assessment processes, offering an inroad to understanding the ways that claimants may find themselves to be at odds with majority ways-of-being specifically within benefits claiming and therefore even more stressed by the process. In Tuck's case, it was also reductive: when Tuck outlined her health timeline on paper, all one could glean was that 'episodes' had happened and that they were 'past.' The written-down timeline on the form was necessarily eliminative, lacking any reference to the intensity/affective dimension contained in the performed version.

Conclusion: effects of the 'How Your Disability Affects You' form

The PIP process relies on sequential chronicity. Moreover, the 'Affects You' form has a speech-text centred chronotope that is segmentable, and ultimately reducible in ways that are very different from the performed productions of Tuck's DEAF way. The integrity of Tuck's deaf-centred ordering could not stand within the rigidity of the paper claim form. The present tense in the title – 'Affects' – that wills the claimant to discuss the impact of disability as it is *now*, frames prior clinical history as merely prologue. It juxtaposes an 'ill' past against a 'well' present-future, which builds upon the narrative that has been constructed over many years of illness being something to get past and move on from. Many lines of enquiry in the 'Affects You' form appear geared towards the individual claimant making a self-affirming statement: she *already has (now)* the ability to live daily life, overcoming any challenges *without* additional personal, technical, or financial support. This admission at once proclaims the claimant to be a capable human, a 'well' being. She in the same instant also proves herself (the claimant) to be too independent to be eligible for funding support. It renders the claimant complicit in the construction of an argument either (a) for her incapacity to function as an adult or (b) that will serve as testimony for the refutation of her claim for funding support.

This sketches why, governed by rules of English textual expressions of history and time the 'Affects You' form can be particularly problematic for DEAF modes of expression. I believe that this was what Tuck attempted to address when she was *'thinking in English.'* It was her method to prove *my mind is ordered like yours. I am well.* In actuality, it was DEAF-centred authoring that enabled me as listener-witness to grapple with the gravity of the impact of her long-term adverse effects. The proofs emerged in the time and rhythm of the 5D telling; the proof must be specific to that particular telling. As Tedlock concludes in his analysis of transcriptions of Zuni myths, the absence of the dynamics of 'telling' in a textual record of a transient utterance is reductive and eliminative of relevant information (1971:127). Without the vitality of the act of performance, the dynamics of telling-the-message are no longer those of the teller, but instead reflect the interpretation of the listener. As Tuck and other DEAF clients at the advisory centre performed their timelines for the 'Affects You' form, I felt I should completely adjust the way the form works to fit DEAF ways of being and expressing, otherwise their testimonies would not fit to the form. However, adjusting the form would place the claimant at risk of being out of step with the metrics used to assess PIP eligibility. So instead the claimant had to fit the form – flattened to match the predetermined sections.

As I watched Tuck climb in and out of her moments of varying mental health, the days and the nights, reconfiguring each instant's impacts, I realised that fitting the message to the form meant removal of Tuck from her own story, her intensity dimension absent in my English re-telling. BSL grammar, exemplified by Tuck's experience of the PIP claims process, is incommensurate with textual English. It is incompatible with institutional formats because 'the particular [language] environment organises a particular regime of language, a regime which incapacitates individuals' (Blommaert 2005:198). These moving, signing, affected bodies become matter out of place (Douglas 1966) because they cannot be witnessed directly by the adjudicators of the PIP benefit. Meanwhile the written-spoken language, and the rigidity of filling in boxes, becomes matter imposed.

Because provability is required due to interpretations of UK equality legislation, the success of a PIP claim ultimately comes down to how convincingly one person can prove the emotionally driven symptoms that disability tolls both within individual experience and also on the society around her. People who are classified as disabled and those who represent them must convincingly argue that the ineffable is palpable, that adverse effects of disabilities are things not only witnessable, but that may also sit within the body as sure as musculature and sinew. And yet, '[p]henomenologically, we are continually caught on the cusp, as it were, between what can and cannot be conceptually grasped, causally explained, or verbally captured' (Jackson 2015:294). Though this ungraspable kernel is precisely the 'stuff' that the 'How Your Disability Affects You' form seeks to capture, validate, and quantify, it does so in a way entirely foreign to the bodily and social context within which Tuck experiences her life.

To paraphrase Barthes, transcription in any setting is 'castratory' because it removes the body from the text (Barthes 2009), the 'grain' from the voice. Written elucidations of sign language remove not only the text, but also deaf people themselves from their own messages. This severing of the body from its voice is a methodological concern that cuts to the very heart of proving *long-term adverse effect*. Tuck's bodied 5D narration and its failure to fit into the 'How Your Disability Affects You' various forms offers an introduction to the ways that deaf people may find themselves at odds with majority ways of engaging with British institutional requirements. Form-fillers have a high degree of responsibility in conferring un-capturable, ineffable elements, and ultimately conveying the claimant's bodied responses as accurately as possible on the paper form. In the end, it is, therefore, this process of applying for PIP that reveals the greatest long-term adverse effects of disability: the emotional and physical impacts of the condition as these emerge in these most complex of communicative webs and the inability in this case to bear witness directly, rather than through a third party.

References

Act, E. (2010). Equality Act 2010: The Explanatory Notes (c. 15).

Barthes, Roland (2009). *The Grain of the Voice: Interviews 1962–1980*. Chicago: Northwestern University Press.

Bechter, Frank Daniel (2009). Of deaf lives: Convert culture and the dialogic of ASL storytelling. PhD Thesis, University of Chicago, Department of Anthropology.

Blommaert, Jan (2005). *Discourse: A Critical Introduction*. Cambridge: Cambridge University Press.

Blommaert, Jan (2015). Chronotopes, scales, and complexity in the study of language in society. *Annual Review of Anthropology* 44:105–116.

Chumley, Lily (2017). Qualia and ontology: Language, semiotics, and materiality; an introduction. *Signs and Society* 5(S1):S1–S20.

Douglas, Mary (1966). *Purity and Danger: An Analysis of Concepts of Pollution and Taboo*. London: Routledge and Keegan Paul.

DWP. 2013 'How Your Disability Affects You'. Accessed 21 March 2018. https://www.gov.uk/government/uploads/system/uploads/attachment_data/file/584199/pip2-how-your-disability-affects-you-form.

DWP (2015). Personal independence payment: The claimant journey. gov.uk/dwp/pip-toolkit.

Gulliver, Michael Stuart (2009). DEAF space, a history: The production of DEAF spaces emergent, autonomous, located and disabled in 18th and 19th century France. PhD Thesis, University of Bristol.

'How Your Disability Affects You'. Accessed 21 March 2018. www.gov.uk/government/uploads/system/uploads/attachment_data/file/584199/pip2-how-your-disability-affects-you-form.PDF.

Jackson, Michael and Albert Piette (Eds.) (2015). *What Is Existential Anthropology?* New York: Berghahn Books.

Kidd, Ian James and Havi Carel (2017). Epistemic injustice and illness. *Journal of applied Philosophy* 34(2):172–190.

Labov, William (1984). Intensity. In D. Schriffin (Ed.), *Meaning, Form and Use in Context: Linguistic Applications*. Washington, DC: Georgetown University Press, 43–70.

Ladd, Paddy (2003). *Understanding Deaf Culture: In Search of Deafhood*. Bristol: Multilingual Matters Ltd.

Parliamentary Review (2018). PIP and ESA [Employment Support Allowance] assessments: claimant experiences. Accessed https://publications.parliament.uk/pa/cm201719/cmselect/cmworpen/355/355.pdf.

Stokoe, William C. (1980) Sign language structure. *Annual Review of Anthropology* 9(1):365–390.

Tedlock, Dennis (1971). On the translation of style in oral narrative. *The Journal of American Folklore* 84(331):114–133.

Wilson, Deirdre and Dan Sperber (2012). *Meaning and Relevance*. Cambridge: Cambridge University Press.

Part III
Health publics

10 On becoming a vegetable

Life, nature, and healing for a hylozoic cult

Roland Littlewood

The community of the Earth People lies above the northern cliffs of the island of Trinidad facing towards Tobago.[1] Its centre is the old wooden house of a long-deserted hamlet, together with some added 'African' huts. For about half a mile in each direction, the secondary bush and scrub of the seasonal rain forest has been cleaned and a variety of trees and perennial cultigens are grown: medicine bushes; trees and plants for cordage and wrapping, and for baskets and calabashes; timber for building; plantain and banana; roots like cassava, sweet potatoes, dasheen, yam, and tannia; aubergine, pineapple, tomato, pigeon peas, callaloo, okra, Indian corn, pumpkin, ginger, sugar cane, and christophene; trees bearing oranges, grapefruit, guava, nuts, mango, avocado, pawpaw, pomerac, tamarind, and breadfruit; garlic and bushes with pepper, shadobenny, and other herbs. Above the settlement, reaching into the lower reaches of the mountains of Trinidad's northern range, are cocoa and coffee, cannabis and tobacco. In the nearby bush grow cress and watermelon, mauby bark, mammy apple, passion fruit, star apple, nutmeg and soursop, whilst along the coast are coconut and almond. The variety of their crops, virtually every Trinidad food plant, justifies the boast of the Earth People that they are indeed living in the original Eden.

Each new member has taken a vegetable or 'fruit name' like Breadfruit, Coconut, Cassava, or Pumpkin;[2] doing so, they say: 'All of we be she [Mother Earth's] fruits.' From 1975, when she gave birth to twins in a remote bush hut along the Trinidad shore, their leader, Jeanette MacDonald (Mother Earth) experienced a series of dramatic revelations and came to understand that the Christian teaching of God the Father as creator was false and that the world was rather the work of a primordial Mother, whom she identified with Nature and with the Earth. Nature had given birth to a race of Black people, but her rebellious Son (the Christian God) re-entered his Mother's

---

1 Ethnographic present tense for 1981–1982.
2 Other names include Pomme Cythère, Eddoes, Dasheen, Tania, Cocorite, Moco, Bodi, Pumpkin Colley, Cane, Orange, Zabocca, Corn, Melangine, and Mango Rose. My adopted name was Tomato [Red Skin], that of my daughter, Letice, was Lettuce, and my wife became Cressels (Cress): all *short* (or supposedly 'new', European) crops.

womb to steal Her power of generation – Life – and thus was able to create the Europeans. These Whites, the Race of the Son/Sun, then enslaved the Blacks and have continued to exploit them. The Way of the Son is the way of Science – of cities, clothes, schools, factories, and wage labour. The Way of The Mother is the Way of Nature – the simplicity of the original Beginning, a simplicity of nakedness and dirt, cultivation of the land by hand and with respect, and of gentle and non-exploiting human relationships.

The woman Jeanette herself is a partial incarnation of The Mother who will fully enter into her Flesh only at the imminent End. Her task at the time of my initial stay with the group in the 1980s was to facilitate the return to Nature by organising the community known as Hell Valley, and to prepare for a Return to the Beginning by teaching her people, The Mother's Children. She has to combat the false doctrines of existing religions which place the Son over the Mother, and to correct the distorted teaching of the Bible, which represents her as the Devil. She stands for Nature and Life in opposition to Science and Death. As the Devil, she is opposed to churches and prisons, education and money, contemporary morals and fashionable opinions. The exact timing of the End is uncertain, but it will be soon and certainly to be expected in Jeanette's physical lifetime. The End will occur through the Whites' environmental destruction or by nuclear war, and by the planet Sun coming nearer to the Earth. As Mother Earth told me: 'Then Time will end, the dead will be raised and the leper cleansed, sickness be healed, the dumb talk, the lame walk, the deaf hear, the blind see, and the [surviving, African descended] Nation speak one language.'

Mother Earth's original revelations ceased in 1976 after she burned all her young family's clothes, household possessions, and Bible in an episode now called The Miracle, through which she brought the sun closer to the earth, thus initiating the Beginning of the End; she tells me: 'I cast my two hands together and I bring [the sun] down between my legs.' At this time, her family were still living with her in the old house, and they were soon joined by an assortment of inquiring young men, generally old friends and neighbours from the capital Port-of-Spain 50 miles away. Her ideas were now debated and consolidated in reflection and debate. She continued to have visions in her dreams, but these were similar to those of other members: premonitions and answers to immediate organisational problems. Normative behaviour in the group reflects the original visions, later chance events, and subsequent deliberation in the community. While around 60 individuals have been active Earth People at different times, in October 1981, 22 were resident in the Valley, predominantly young adult males, with perhaps 20 sympathisers and occasional members in town. There were annual naked marches into Port-of-Spain, which sometimes ended in arrests, together with occasional raids on the settlement by police and social workers, who placed the younger children in an orphanage (from which some managed to escape back to the Valley). In opposition to what they call the *material* world,[3] the Earth People all go naked, sleeping out on the bare ground, and maintaining themselves through fishing and cultivation of the land using only cutlasses and axes. In describing how residents of the valley take the names of vegetables, and how they engage with other 'Natural' materials of the Earth, this chapter explores how the floating significance of 'Life,' and the affronts to 'Life,' emerge from the materiality of the valley of the Earth People and normative Trinidadian society. 'Life' is a totallising concept for the people of the Valley, imminently present in the Earth herself, and a degree of ambivalence arises in relation to nature. Death, disease, and disharmony arise when the objects of nature are 'tapped' by the energies of the *material*(istic), non-natural world. This type of 'tapping' is not intentional; it is simply the inevitable outcome of the affordances of the material world. To what extent do members of the Valley consider themselves part of the extra-human physical world? To take a vegetable name is more than just an affirmation of joining the group: it is a recognition that the individual is now more part of the natural world, the Earth, than are other human beings. All the physical world is alive – it is Life. Even a stone, to an extent, is alive, less alive perhaps than a plant which can grow or an animal which can move,[4] but nevertheless alive in a similar way. A stone or piece of ground has agency, and adverse local climatic events are attributed by the Earth People to the industrial removal of petroleum – the blood of the earth – and such removal is answered in angry injury. At the same time, the group is contemptuous of local magical practices and sorcery, not because of the moral dimension but simply because they could not be effective, the practitioner having a too concrete notion of the association of human action and physical material. When I told the Dominican priests in their presbytery down the coast about this, they agreed that the Earth People were in many ways more 'modern' than their own parishioners in the villages.

So what actually happens when a young townsman joins the group and takes a vegetable or fruit name? There is no sudden transformation. As a man of African descent, he is already more part of nature and life than

3 The English word 'material' is not used by the Earth People to refer to the physical world but to the social world of the Son (God): as Mother Earth punningly puts it: 'Women thinks more materialise. And men are more Natural. That is what I am seeing here in the country . . . And that is really the spirit [of God] because the spirit try to hold the mothers more, because knowing that the mothers is the Spirit of the Earth, well then, he must have them more confused. Too much of dressing, too much of material.' Compare this with the prevalent local attitude as described by Miller (1994). Throughout, *material* in italics is the local concept as described by Mother Earth, and material (not in italics) is the analytical concept.

4 They are hylozoic rather than pantheistic. The latter still implicates a two-memberedness of (a) divinity dwelling in, (b) the material. I take 'hylozoic' to mean that the physical has an inherent quality of life, the idea being non-transcendent. Divinity – in this case, Mother Earth's divinity – is identical with Life itself in the physical world: there is no distinction between 'natural' and 'supernatural' (cf. Durkheim 1976 [1912]:26–31).

others (and more than women) might be, and the vegetable name acknowledges his conscious acceptance of this. Other Black Trinidadians, particularly women, now generally tend towards European urban ways.[5] The recruit does not take on any particular characteristics of the vegetable, thus one called Lime, would not be particularly 'sour,' although the initial choice of the name may be suggested by physical appearance, for Bodi (bean) is tall and lanky. Nor is subsequent behaviour judged by the plant identity or related back to it. Quite simply, all become generically 'she fruits.' It is more than a name, it is the recognition of being part of Nature.

The exact extent to which we are inherently part of Nature, part of Life, is of no especial interest to the group. It suffices to simply be here and to be working towards a more natural Life. As Tania sings:

> *You know, uh*
> *They know, as well as the doctors know, uh, uh*
> *The lawyers know*
> *As well as the President know*
> *Oh that is Life, uh*
> *The Earth is Life*
> *Sing it loud, Sing it loud,*
> *I know, Yeh, uh*
> *You know, uh*
> *They know, yeh*
> *As well as the professors know, uh*
> *The preachers know*
> *As well as the children in the town know,*
> *The Earth is Life, the Earth is Life*
> *Sing it loud, Sing it loud, uh*
> *The children are feeding from the Earth now, uh*
> *They cannot do without it . . .*

To be inherently part of Nature makes some decisions easier for the Earth people in terms of how to live one's life, but there is still the possibility of voluntary backsliding, and a conscious decision to work harder for the group is valued. Mother Earth told me:

> *Some of them that come, comes with a spirit of seeing themselves an'*
> *working the land. Some come, they want to play. They not really think-*
> *ing of what they're doing so then they usually leave because working*
> *they find that too hard to do. So they don't stay, they leave. But those*
> *who stay they go through little cutses, biteses you know, and fight up*

---

5 After some months with the group, I was regarded as only 'White on the outside' but really Black 'inside' in contradistinction to the average Trinidadian: Black outside but White inside.

with it. When people comes to the bush, since I am living here, I watch them go, they would lie down on the ground there looking at the ground to see if it is clean or dirty. [Others] they just threw themselves down: 'oh it is nice.' The Spirit [of God] know it's the End so the more that he can get the Flesh to play, you know, they wouldn't want the Beginning. This is it all. The more you can get them material-like, more food, more party, they wouldn't want to stay in the bush . . . it ain't me to change them. They got to change side. They must know Left from Right. This is the fight – from Right to Left.[6] Life.

The centrality of the concept of 'Life' within the practice of the Earth People, and its all-encompassing implications, such that, as Tania sings 'the Earth is Life,' allows for a deeper investigation of what 'Life' – and indeed what 'Earth' – is.

Is Life, then, a 'floating signifier'?

The Earth People's use of the term 'Life' as referring to whole of emergent Nature, and thus of everything, suggests Life and Nature and divinity cannot be empirically separated. Everything is alive, though not to the same extent. Social anthropologists have been recurrently interested in the cognitive implications of such local ideas as *mana, baraka, tapu, orenda,* and *mangu*: categories which Lévi-Strauss (1951:xlix, l), in his introduction to a collection of Mauss' essays, characterises as 'floating signifiers' *(significants flottants)* with their *valeur symbolique zero*. Often referred to in English as 'empty signifiers' or 'empty concepts,' these very inchoate ideas, however central for a particular society, are not easily glossed either by locals or by anthropologists. The more you look for the particular to which one refers, the more the concept disintegrates. It is everywhere, yet nowhere in particular. Is *baraka* in North Africa a saintly disposition? Or a power? Or is it a healing process or health itself, success or luck, piety or character, fertility or virility? Is it inherited, earned, learned or a gift from God? All these and more (Crapanzano 1973).

Boyer (1986), in his critique of attempts to define more exactly certain of these categories, refers to them as 'mana-terms' following Mauss' and Durkheim's reliance on Codrington's (1891) Melanesian data. 'Mana is ethnographically unavoidable,' argues Holbraad (2007:189). Powerful social organising concepts that can perhaps be seen as such from the outside, they seem untranslatable, 'virtually meaningless, yet are placed at the centre of traditional discourse' and have been commonly translated as a 'vital force'

---

6 That they are politically 'left' is not lost on them, but the original Left/Right distinction comes from surviving fragments from the Burning and from Jeanette's stronger left eye. Handshakes are left-handed, and a common greeting is 'All Left!'.

or a mystical energy (Boyer 1986:50), the very paradigm of magic (Mauss 1904). Keesing (1985) argues that anthropologists have traditionally reified these terms as if they were metaphysical entities rather than what they probably are – metaphors for social relationships. Local informants can talk about the effects of a mana-term, its personnel and consequences, but they cannot readily categorise it; one can perhaps see what an empty signifier *does*, but not what it *is*. In Melanesia, say Mauss (1904), *mana* has served as a force, a being, a substance, a state, an action, a quality. It is *mana* that gives things social, material, and spiritual weight; serves as property and wealth; it kills, creates magical objects, and endows spirits; it is the force of sickness and fertility; the power of a magician or rite; the source of all efficacy and life; of action at a distance but also of the ether (Mauss 1904); and it may involve a 'physical shock which may be compared to the effect of an electrical discharge' (Durkheim 1912:190).

Against structuralist arguments that cosmologies concretise general use terms (which can be used to fill in gaps in the cosmological framework) and intellectualist explanations (that these terms serve as implicit theoretical principles that explain certain effects in the natural and social worlds), Boyer proposes instead a closer look at the different registers of use of each term, distinguishing for instance between particular expertise and general gossip. And Holbraad (2007) argues for a fluid conception of a similar Afro-Cuban category, *aché*, as both material and transcendent.

In this chapter, we are concerned less with any general characteristics (if such there could be) of these ideal categories of the human mind than with noting two aspects: (a) that the contemporary Western world uses apparently similar terms, particularly in the areas of physics and therapeutics, and (b) these concepts are generally embodied in individual experience and social action. It is likely that the anthropological focus on small-scale communities with their own particular 'floating signifier' has ignored the fact that certain English terms, both personal and impersonal, not only general cosmological principles but also the explanation of personal fortune, illness, and other contingencies – are remarkably similar: but now outside the apparent area of what we once called the 'sacred.' In attempts to understand the traditional terms, ethnographers have frequently glossed their use by parallels drawn from physics, notably power, energy, and action at a distance. What they have perhaps ignored is the use of these very terms in Western societies, in practical everyday situations and in systems of healing, which inform particular individual circumstances, and yet are informed by abstracted theoretical cosmologies (and, indeed, can be understood as abstracted cosmologies themselves). An obvious therapeutic example is the common use of 'energy' as a medico-therapeutic-spiritual idiom (Littlewood and Reynolds 2018).

The Earth People ridicule customary ideas of impurity, but their values generate their own recognition of what, for want of a better term, we may term 'pollution,' for they avoid clothes and tinned and packaged food and meat and deprecated my use of a notebook and the use of menstrual tampons (Mother Earth merely stuffs a rag between her thighs). These material technologies are seen as disgusting and are certainly a serious risk to life. Cure for illness caused by urban life are quite simply to leave the town and join the valley's Culture of the Body. At the same time, they share the local villagers' ideas about common ailments and use local plant tisanes for medicine.

The Earth People frequently are stung by scorpions and are encouraged to eat earth as a remedy – a local practice – but, not always with success:

JAKATAN: *I bit by a scorpion and the first thing I study is eat dirt.*
RL: *Did you?*
J [LAUGHING]: *No.*
MOTHER EARTH [reproachfully]: *Is you self talking there and you leave it out.*
J: *I figure I got enough Life.*

Dirt is Nature and Life; as Mother Earth explained:

> *When I smell myself, I was something else! I smell very awful, I what they call 'awful until that scent wear out' and I start smelling normal – what is dirt. We don't study bathing: if your body too clean, the pores open and disease get in. Your skin come off in layers as you wash. You must keep it on as a protection. In the city the more clean the children the more sick they get. In a too clean house the children dig dirt out of the boards and eat it. It is part of the Culture of the Body. Sickness develop as different parts of diseases in the body: too much is chemical. So then you a become a machine instead of a human.*

The Earth People are opposed to hospitals and biomedicine, and Mother Earth refused some pharmaceuticals I brought her for her own congestive cardiac failure although she accepted some *racket* (prickly pear cactus). Local bush medicine is regarded as purely physical and natural. It works just because of its inherent properties – and is the same stuff as pharmaceutical medicine, although in smaller and less dangerous quantities. Name, colour, and shape of plant have no association with its healing qualities, it is purely that it is Earth.

Nature in Trinidad

Trinidad's history is not atypical of the British Caribbean: conquest from Spain, the development of the agro-industrial sugar plantations by slave labour (which, political historians have argued, was the model for the European industrial factory), and the emancipation of the slaves in 1838, followed by the introduction of indentured labourers from India; the collapse of the price of cane sugar after the loss of colonial preference and competition with European beet sugar; the collapse of the other main exports, coffee and cocoa; universal adult suffrage in 1946; increasing local participation in Legislative Council progressing to internal self-government in the 1950s, and independence in 1962 as a single parliamentary state with the neighbouring island of Tobago. Trinidad differs from other West Indian islands in its relative wealth from oil and its low population density (despite continued immigration during the nineteenth and twentieth centuries from the smaller islands). Relations between Africans, Indians, and the small European population may be said to be comparatively relaxed if not altogether harmonious and practical social segregation based on 'colour' lasted well after independence. Colour, class, and poverty still run together.

Trinidad's oil resources (off-shore wells and refining industry) have been intensively exploited since independence. Together with natural gas deposits in the southeast and the world's largest pitch lake near the western town of San Fernando, they are the basis for the national economy through taxation on the international corporations and partial nationalisation. Tourism has not developed (except at carnival time), perhaps because of the scarcity of beaches, but also because it was once seen as politically demeaning for the country. The local standard of living is high, reputedly the third highest in the Americas after the US and Canada; in 1981, there was one motor vehicle for every ten of the island's 1.2 million population and, a few rural areas excepted, concrete houses, electricity, television, healthcare, piped water, and metalled roads were taken for granted by all – the labour intensive agricultural cultivation of sugar, coffee, cocoa, and ground provisions has been effectively abandoned, and in 1981, Trinidad became a net importer of sugar. Meat, dairy products, and flour have always been imported, but now the foreign exchange surplus allowed the bulk of local food to be brought in from abroad, rice from Guyana and ground provisions from the smaller and poorer islands of the Lesser Antilles.

In cosmopolitan post-war Trinidad, 'agriculture was linked with backwardness and degradation . . . agricultural was what you wanted escape from' (Naipaul 1985:78). The local villagers who still produce some local provisions for village consumption generally deplore this, as do their relatives in town who say they return frequently to their natal villages for fresh air and good food, at the same time as they criticise the government for abandoning the rural areas – 'Behind God's back.' Many of the local older Creole-speaking inhabitants regret the depopulation of the coast and the passing of traditional rural life. Whilst valuing the benefits of electricity, piped water, and pensions, they criticise the young men's expectations of an easy life. They say of the new generation, 'It come so all they want is fêting. They can't take hard work again.' They afford grudging respect to the return to agricultural life in Hell Valley all the more so as the Earth People come from Port of Spain, Trinidad's capital city, and a centre of metropolitan life in the West Indies. Village opinions about Trinidad's future often echo that of the Earth People: that the removal of the oil, the blood of the soil, is slowly turning the land into an unproductive arid desert. The earth is not a limitless resource. They too are suspicious of the newer farming techniques advocated by the government agricultural officers and, refusing pesticides or fertilisers, continue to plant and harvest according to the phases of the moon. The oil wealth, they say, is temporary: it will disappear, leaving Trinidadians now unable to plant, starving in their once fertile but now 'unbalanced' land. But for now, argues Jobie, a local fisherman in Pinnaclo village, 'If you can't buy rice, you just pick a plantain. The earth is the mother for true!' A number of the younger village men demonstrate an allegiance to Rastafari through wearing dreadlocks and have some knowledge of Jamaican Rasta ideas. They have remained behind in the village, as opposed to migrating to the city, to pursue a *natural* life and they express considerable sympathy for the Earth People. Two of them told me that they would actually join the group if not for the Earth People's practice of nudity and for Mother Earth's reputation for making everybody work so hard. Some of them meet the Earth People in the bush, smoke a little ganja with them, and offer the fish they have caught in their nets in exchange for ground provision. Itinerant preachers, passing prophets, and the numerous founders of small short-lived sects see in the Earth People some justification for their own beliefs. They are disconcerted on actual contact. A local preacher who had a vision went to the valley. Mother Earth summarised the encounter, saying, 'He said, "Here is Eden!" I said, "You right!" Then he say, "Armageddon going to come the next week." I say, "You are wrong," and he fuss and he carry on and he pass on.' Rural Catholic priests, faced with declining church attendance, privately envy the fervour and discipline in the Valley of Decision.

From arcadia to utopia

'The earth was not made purposely for you to be lords of it, and we to be your slaves, servants and beggars;' says Gerrard Winstanley in his 1649 *A Declaration From the Poor Oppressed People of England*, 'but it was made to be a common livelihood to all, without respect of persons' (Winstanley 1973:99). One of the sources of our Western counter-current lay in the mediaeval peasant of arcadia of Cockaigne, the fairy tale, topsy-turvy land where there exists a natural abundance of food but no oppressive nobility or interfering lawyers. In this poor man's heaven, 'al[l] is commun to young and old,/to stoute and sterne, me[e]k and bold' (Morton 1922:18). The early modern representation of this alimentary paradise (together with its herbal remedies, wise women, astrologers, almanacks, and celestial signs) seems associated with what Hobsbawm (1959) has termed the 'pre-political response' of social bandits and popular outlaws, of ludic and transvestite Luddites rebelling against changes from above, in an aggressive levelling of the traditional enemies of the poor – prelates, lawyers, land surveyors, foreigners, dealers – in a dramatic but futile attempt to regenerate a stable agrarian peasant society.

Maurice and Jean Bloch (1980) have noted that our word 'nature' carries in contemporary Europe four associated meanings: the chronologically pre-social, an internal bodily process, the universal and inevitable order of the organic and inorganic, and (perceived or imagined) 'primitive' peoples (Bloch 1977). All find resonances in Mother Earth's pre-existent and elemental domain of the Mother of the Nation (see Littlewood 1993:5, 80). Such an arcadia is a rather comfortable and cheerful place recalling the sylvan liberties of Cockaigne and Arden, the domicile of the wild men and Robin Hood in the Tudor masques, rather than the grim wilderness of Judaeo-Christianity in which man comes across God only in brief and arduous encounters. 'Mother Nature' recalls us to a bountiful Merrie England, not the Sinai desert.

For the classical Greeks, the Earth emanating out of chaos, had been a sensate organism. Usually personified as female, she was the ultimate origin of all, and the various Hellenistic cults of the Great Mother acknowledged her as the active and fundamental source of our being. By contrast, in the Latin tradition, the Old Testament God, who got around to creating the Earth only on the third day, kept her firmly in a subordinate position, for had he not conjured her *ex nihilo*? A 'Mother Earth' did survive in Latin and post-Reformation Christianity, like the planets of the pagans, but unlike their gods, an Earth of somewhat undifferentiated matter rather than volition, which awaited arousal and impregnation by a man formed in God's image. As Simone de Beauvoir puts it, 'the husbandman marvelled at the mystery of the fecundity that burgeoned in his furrows and in the maternal body' – a sleeping fecundity that required awakening and then control (de Beauvoir 1972:99). Mother Nature had lost her primacy; in the mediaeval cosmos, Man and Nature remained distinct but associated through the dominion given to Man by a transcendent deity. The land was not to be supplicated but subjugated, ordered, for 'every moving thing that liveth shall be meat for you' (Genesis 9:3).

By contrast, to quote the Ranters:

> When we die we shall be swallowed up into the infinite spirit as a drop into the ocean and so be as we were; and if ever we be raised again, we shall rise a horse, a cow, a root, a flower and such like.
>
> (Thomas 1984:138)

The Familists and Giordano Bruno too had asserted that a Mother Nature rather than a God still governed the world, but the new mechanical science of the Renaissance offered rather a continued domination over a divinely ordered world, leading Man to 'Nature with all her children to bind her to your service and make her your slave,' to Bacon's 'truly masculine birth of time [in which man] would conquer and subdue Nature, to shake her to her foundations' (Bacon 1964). Mother Nature was to be first stripped naked and then penetrated by Man; the Royal Society promised its male scientists that 'The Beautiful Bosom of Nature will be Exposed to our view. . . . We shall enter its Garden, and taste of its Fruits and satisfy ourselves with its plenty' (cited in Easlea 1980:129, 217–18). Something not so very different remains the everyday view of Nature in urban Trinidad. Nineteenth-century Trinidad, Donald Wood notes, was 'bewitched' with notions of boundless fertility; at the abolition of slavery, only one-thirtieth of the land was under cultivation (Wood 1968:24–25, 19). While members of the revolutionary commune in Naipaul's novel *Guerrillas* (1975) seem to parallel some of the arguments of Mother Earth herself – 'All revolutions begin with the land. Men are born on the earth, every man has his one spot, it is his birth-right' (Naipaul 1976:17) – their suggestion that one gains one's identity through cultivating the fertile soil does not immediately evoke everyday Trinidadian resonances. Rather, urban Trinidadians feel attached to the soil by default: they would be elsewhere if they could, for the land now seems marginal to the real life of London, New York, or even Port-of-Spain. Though rural self-sufficiency is sometimes economically necessary as a springboard or failsafe, it is hardly the ultimate goal.

Both Mother Earth and Naipaul's fictional guerrillas draw less on the rural Trinidadian peasant's prosaic attitude to the earth than on urban and Romantic notions of a hypostasised Nature. The very word *nature* is seldom used in Trinidad English except in the sense of sexual desire, particularly that of men,

> supporting nature is like taking a long sweet drink: you will just drink and go on so. You take as much as your appetite can take. Like a man is married and his wife start have children he has to go outside to get something to satisfy his nature.
>
> (Kerr 1952:87)

Although its other meanings are recognised, Mother Earth's alternative name of 'Mother Nature' only occasionally causes a snigger. *Nature* in Trinidad is something inevitable and independent of conscious will; to restrain it is dangerous. It is not just the sexual impulse itself but the very inevitability of conception manifest in the number of children a woman is predetermined to bear: an inevitability which can be countered only through a self-defeating, 'respectable' but arid, choice between contraception and abstinence.

The Romantics' cultivation of Nature transformed the ascetic vision of the walled New Jerusalem into a fertile garden, and the pilgrim into a gardener. 'When I was in my earthly garden a-digging with my spade,' said the mystic Roger Crab, 'I saw into the Paradise of God from whence my father Adam was cast forth' (Thomas 1984:237). In the eighteenth century, 'nature cults' – Martinism, Masonry, Theophilanthropy – proliferated together with the artificial Arcadia of landscape gardening; the end of topiary presaged the end of swaddling, for the child was to be cultivated in its nursery as a tender plant. Like the Earth People, the children of the French Revolution took the names of fruits; to 'culture' implied natural growth and organic continuity rather than the inculcating of rigid and artificial institutions. Man could not, however, completely surrender to Nature for he still planted and plundered her: the urban gardener's vision of a vanished Eden was only a nostalgic pastiche, and the Liberty Tree just a maypole. Mediaeval Latin Christianity, mechanical science, and Romanticism alike allowed that Man could dominate the rest of creation 'out there.' Even the Ranter pantheist had to deal with the problem of what was going on when he ate a plant (a transformation within Nature?), and whether that was any less significant than if he ate an animal or, indeed, another human.

The same question emerges in Hell Valley. If all is Nature, why is it somehow less appropriate to kill an animal for meat than to cultivate and eat a plant? The Earth People certainly have a notion of a 'weed.' While their clearing of the apparently undifferentiated bush to bring forth cultivated crops can be seen simply as transformations and reorganisations within Nature, their refusal to eat animals argues for some residual Natural hierarchy. To gather rather than to cultivate is certainly an option for the hardline vegetarian – like those Doukhobors who said they could live on fruit and honey (Scott 2017) – but the very notion of gathering itself demonstrates some hierarchy within Nature; pantheism, if pursued to one logical end, might include meat eating, perhaps even cannibalism. If all such ingestions are merely transformations in an essentially undifferentiated domain, the way lies freely open to amoral antinomianism. This particular logical difficulty (and utopians are the most determined of logicians) has led many groups to alternate, as with sexuality, between a rigorous asceticism and a thoroughgoing antinomianism.

William Blake did not regard what we may term 'Romantic gardening' as simply recognising Man's place in Nature: 'As of old now anew began Babylon again in Infancy, call'd Natural Religion' (Blackstone 2015; 209). Blake, a decided phenomenologist, objected to the idea that Nature was something external which could be apprehended independently of our self-consciousness. She is a projection of us and thus 'Everything that lives is Holy' (ibid: 42). Rousseau solved the problem rather differently when he distinguished the Natural from the Social as two rather different types of knowledge and being. Man was both Social (in his institutions) and Natural (in his bodily feelings); in the *Discourse on Equality*, he tends to argue a preference for the latter, but in *The Social Contract*, he accepts an interplay between the Social and Natural. This distinction between Nature as a type of undifferentiated stuff and bodily experience, contrasted with the Social as mental organisation and institution, leads us from radical Puritanism to contemporary social science, and to socialism; from cyclical returns to a linear unfolding in evolutionary time. The remaining millennialists have continued to see Nature and Society as distinct but comparable domains of the same type of established order.

Whatever the logical snares – whether they regarded God as in His garden, as part of the garden itself, or as altogether outside it – the radical counter-current deployed an idea of Nature to demonstrate the artificiality and unreality of existing social institutions. Whether we take its communities as atavistically harking back to come lost peasant Arcadia or as radically new utopian institutions, they were conceived in a harmony with a physical world which embraced all things, a harmony which was already demonstrated by the tribal peoples. A common conclusion was that land could not really be owned; along with Rousseau and Winstanley, the counter-current argued that human alienation and inequality are rooted alike in property.[7] The Shakers taught that North American Indians had a superior religion to Christianity precisely because it was not rooted in a capitalist exploitation of nature (Nordhoff 1966:235).

Taps as anti-Life

The Earth People are not theologians and are more concerned with practice than doctrine. Is Life, then, a fairly empty term merely signifying common African ancestry, the nature that surrounds us and our relative aspirations? You can have more or less of it and gather it by living in the valley, and it is a term of praise for those evidently working harder. It is the power acquired by life in the settlement. Without this being a complete contrary, it is opposed by the *tap*,[8] an act of the Son which connotes a failure of goodwill or determination in the individual, but not causing major accidents or illness; also any inappropriate interference with another member such as eavesdropping, borrowing, or begging; and any bad feelings or jealousy which might drain off the energy of another. This last, affective, use is sometimes subsumed, half-jokingly, under the 1970's hippie term 'bad vibes.' Like the local idea of *maljo* (evil eye) (Littlewood 1993), tapping is not an intended action, and it has to be brought to the surface and ventilated. On one occasion during the wet season, Coconut ('a college boy and should know better!' says Mother Earth), who had a reputation for borrowing tools without permission, took Tannia's axe, and when he eventually returned it, he dumped it on the ground unceremoniously and was publicly reprimanded by Mother Earth. The next day, Tannia took his axe and whilst felling wet timber, he slipped and cut his foot deeply, his first accident in two years. Mother Earth and Breadfruit cleaned the wound and dressed it with cocoa husk scrapings and then rebuked Coconut again. She told him forcefully that his borrowing

---

7 The 'modernists, Winstanley and Rousseau, saw the primary fault as prophets (leading to spiritual alienation); others argued spiritual alienation led to material attenuation.
8 A term which derives from the physical survival of a small metal object after the Burning.

was the cause of the accident. Coconut protested that he had no influence on axes. Everybody who was by, tired of Coconut's habitual borrowing, chorused mockingly 'It your vibes! We saw them going out.' They started laughing, for 'vibes' is a bit of a joke Americanism, and Coconut stormed off in tears. Mother Earth quietened the laughter and told the group, now enlarged by others drifting in to observe the fuss, that Coconut was hurt at the suggestion that he had wanted to hurt Tannia, who then said himself that it was his own fault as he had not secured the axe handle properly. Mother argued that that alone would have not caused the accident but blamed him for lending his tools to people. She then seized the opportunity to offer a long homily to the whole community: ultimately all their accidents were caused by disharmony in the group, particularly people going off to the *high woods* to grow their private supply of ganja.

So *Life* and *Vibes* do not operate in complete independence of human choice and intention. And Mother Earth's own role mixes the physically human and the 'divine,' or ultimate, course. The partial incarnation and the premorchial mother in the human Jeanette seems obviously modelled on the Christian God's Incarnation in the human Jesus.[9] As she says:

> *I am not completely myself as yet. I am here, half of me out here and half still to enter the Flesh. When I am completely myself then I have more work to do. . . . I will be having all powers. So I am trying to show my people what it will be like when the hour comes for the Beginning.*

She is not regarded as a celestial person, but rather with warm, affectionate feelings as their Mother, almost as if she were the human mother of this whole family. There is no sacred text for the group – whose origin and continuation lie solely in her personality, as charisma. It is Mother who relates everyday events to their central purpose, and it is in her that the awesome power of Life will finally be made manifest. Her mood is quickly reflected in the feeling of the day: if she feels unwell, the Earth People are subdued; if lively, they are filled with new energy and confidence. Her usual station is by the central cooking area. Shouts of 'Mother want you' are quickly relayed to those working away from the household and are immediately obeyed. Her critical comments on the progress of the cooking, the tidiness of the men's house, or on general moral are listened to with quiet attention, and her wishes carried out. At the same time, this is done with much cheerful abuse, yelling: 'Ganja now make your mind travel. It not supposed to travel.' Mother Earth is Life, and as the woman moves and her moods

9 In general, sources we might identify for the Earth People's mythology include local Christianity, children's comics, Hollywood 'Sword and Sandal' epics, and international news on the radio and in the popular press. This Mother Earth is an incarnation also of Polyphemus, the natural spirit attacking the male hero Ulysses, the Son.

stir the Valley, Flesh and Life are one. But that same material that gives Life also can be cause for contestation, and the warmth of affection holds an ambivalence. On one occasion, she helped herself to Coconut's calabash. He protested, 'That my own fig [banana].' Breadfruit immediately reproached him: 'That Mother Earth own. All food comes from Mother Earth,' but added to general laughter, 'An' she ai' got no fucking manners.'

Acknowledgements

Part of this text was published in Littlewood 1993. My original fieldwork in Trinidad was funded by the Social Science Research Council with a Post-Doctoral Conversion Fellowship.

References

Bacon, F. (1964). Masculine Birth of Time. In *Philosophy of Francis Bacon*. Trans. Benjamin Farrington Liverpool: Liverpool University Press (cit. n. 6.), 62, 72.

Blackstone, B. (2015). *English Blake*. Cambridge. Cambridge University Press.

Bloch, M (1977). The past and the present in the present. *Man* (n.s.) 12:278–292.

Bloch, M. and J. H. Bloch (1980). Women and the Dialectics of Nature in the Eighteenth-century French Thought. In C. P. MacCormack and M. Strathern (Eds.), *Nature, Culture and Gender*. Cambridge University Press, 25–41.

Boyer, P. (1986). The 'empty' categories of traditional thinking: A semantic and pragmatic description. *Man* (n.s.) 21:50–64.

Crapanzano, V. (1973). *The Hamadsha*. Berkeley University of California Press.

Codrington, R.H. (1891). *The Melanesians* Oxford: Clarendon Press.

de Beauvoir, S. (1972). *The Second Sex*. Harmondsworth: Penguin.

Durkheim, E. (1976 [1912]). *The Elementary Forms of the Religious Life*. London: Allen and Unwin.

Easlea, B. (1980). *Witch Huntings, Magic and the New Philosophy: An Introduction to the Debates of the Scientific Revolution 1450–1750*. Sussex: Harvester.

Hobsbawm, E. J. (1959). *Primitive Rebels: Studies in Archaic Forms of Social Movement in the 19th and 20th Centuries*. Manchester: The University Press.

Holbraad, M. (2007). The Power of Powder: Multiplicity and Motion in the Divinatory Cosmology of Cuban Ifa (or *mana*, again). In C. Henare, M. Holbraad and S. Wastell (Eds.), *Thinking through Things: Theorising Artefacts Ethnographically*. London: Routledge, 189–225.

Keesing, R.M. (1985). Conventional metaphors and anthropological metaphysics. *Journal of Anthropological Research* 41:201–217.

Kerr, M. (1952). *Personality and Conflict in Jamaica*. Liverpool: Liverpool University Press.

Lévi-Strauss, C. (1951). Introduction à l'oeuvre de Marcel Mauss. In Mauss (Ed.), *Sociologie et anthropologie*. Paris: Presses.

Littlewood, R. (1993). *Pathology and Identity. The Work of Mother Earth in Trinidad*. Cambridge: Cambridge University Press.

Littlewood, R. and E. Reynolds (2018). The Embodiment of a Floating Signifier (in press, Anthropology and Medicine).

Mauss, M. (1904/1972) *A General Theory of Magic*. London: Routledge and Kegan.

Miller. D. (1994). Style and anthology, In J. Friedman (Ed.), *Consumption and Identity*. Reading: Harwood.

Morton, A. L. (1922). *The English Utopia*. London: Lawrence & Wishart LTD.

Naipaul, V.S. (1985/1984). *Beyond the Dragon's Mouth*. London: Abacus.

Nordhoff, C. (1966/1875). *The Communist Societies of the United States*. New York: Dover.

Scott, A. (2017). *The Promise of Paradise: Utopian Communities in British Columbia*. Pender Harbour, British Columbia. Harbour Publishing.

Smith, N. (Ed.), (2014). *A Collection of Ranter Writings: Spiritual Liberty and Sexual Freedom in the English Revolution*. London: Pluto.

Thomas, K. (1984). *Man and the Natural World: Changing Attitudes in England 1500–1800*. Harmondsworth: Penguin.

Winstanley, G. (1973). *The Law of Freedom and Other Writings*. Ed. C. Hill. Harmondsworth: Penguin.

Wood, D. (1968). *Trinidad in Transition: The Years after Slavery*. Oxford: Oxford University Press.

11 Making the body local

The suburban shitizen

David Jeevendrampillai

It was a cold, wintry Thursday night as the locals poured into one of their favourite bars by the waterfront of the River Thames by the town of Kingston, southwest London. Champagne was popped, spirits were warmed, and I was told – after having a glass of bubbles thrust into my hand – that 'what you can see here, Jeeva' is a 'community that works.' Just a few moments before, in the borough's council chamber, a decision was reached by the planning committee. An application to build luxury flats on the site of disused water filtration beds, which at one time supplied London with much of its clean water – located just a short 20-minute walk up the riverside path in the nearby suburb of Surbiton – had been rejected. For months, members of the Surbiton community had met, discussed, organised, and campaigned to block the application. The beds were built in the 1850s in order to deliver drinking water to London's booming population. The technology was new but went on to form the basis of water filtering systems around the world. The site was used up until the 1970s, after which it became derelict. For the locals, the site held a rich cultural history that linked the suburb to the history of clean water, epidemiology, and modern health and helped make London and Surbiton the places that they are today. Furthermore, owing to being left largely untouched for the best part of 30 years, the site was home to a rich ecology that included the rare Daubenton bat species that feeds on the insects above the still water on the site.

Fast forward a few months. I sit with Tim as the early spring sun dips behind the rusty blue railings of the old filtration site, which we can see across the road from the pub. We have met for an overdue catch up. During my time conducting fieldwork into community building practices in the area, I met Tim regularly, around two or three times a week. However, in the build up to the planning decision, we met less than once a month as Tim cancelled meetings and was relatively distant and unengaged. Now, Tim apologised and told me that, as he looked back, he knew he was not 'in the best place.' He told me how the stress and strain of being a key spokesperson for the community had taken a toll on him physically and mentally. He described how his marriage was under strain due to the amount of time he was spending in community meetings, how he felt he carried the responsibility of the community, and how he was drinking too much. This stress had somatised in his guts, he had developed irritable bowels, and during the council meeting itself, Tim had to run to the bathroom numerous times between giving testimony. The irony was not lost on him that in the act of saving a site to which clean water was traced during the cholera epidemics of the 1850s, he had himself developed dysentery. In his struggle to preserve a historical landmark in the development of the modern city, one that was pivotal in the management of bodily fluids, Tim's body felt the strain.

It is the relationship between the body and the city that I wish to talk about in this chapter. Tim was proud of where he lived. He regularly gave walking tours beside the filter beds and told the story of urban planning, epidemiology, and cholera. This chapter outlines how the modern city emerged through the need to regulate and maintain the health of a population via the management of faecal waste. The city, and the regulatory bodies of urban planning, arose from the development and building of an integrated sewer system that binds the city together. This achievement of Victorian engineering has been celebrated, and it has become a source of pride for Londoners like Tim. Yet, in trying to save its infrastructure, to which his sense of localness is tied, Tim ironically developed health issues around unruly 'shit.' This position, I argue, is symptomatic of the demand made of the modern subject, that they must perform a mode of decent citizenship and appear a citizen that 'works' whilst keeping out of sight the abject material aspects of the ill health that arise from that performance.

Citizenship and the city

Paul Rabinow's *French Modern* (1995) describes how urban planning arose amidst a perceived need to manage and govern populations of cities. Fuelled by urban public health epidemics of cholera and the rise of scientific rationalism, Rabinow outlines how a managerial class of urban experts in the form of town planners and new municipal forms of government served as technologies of power. The management and regulation of populations and cities gave rise to the modern subject and the modern city. Such Foucauldian perspectives on urban planning, whilst important in illuminating the historical contingency of power, have been critiqued as positioning the state in an assumed vertical position of supreme authority, a 'super-coordinator' of the process and institutions of governance (Sharma and Gupta 2006:9). Nikolas Rose (1996) has drawn attention to the role non-state institutions, communities, and individuals play in the mundane process of governance. Such processes have become increasingly important, and within the UK context, the increasing 'de-statization' of government (Rose 1996:56) can be seen in the Localism Act (2011) which aimed to increase the amount of decision-making powers for communities and individuals. Whilst the overriding accompanying narrative from government has been one of increasing inclusion and participation in democracy, this chapter shows how such procedures also place a burden of action onto local communities and particular individuals. Partaking in the urban planning process as a 'local' is, I argue, an act of performing biolegitimacy (following Fassin 2009), a process of demonstrating that one's life, way of life, and – by extension – notions of a good local built environment, are worth maintaining. Biolegitimacy, states Fassin, gives the foundation to 'biological citizenship' (ibid:51), which is a state afforded to a person upon proof of their pathology. For example, Fassin notes the case of a Kenyan man who was living in France under permanent threat of exclusion. Upon a diagnosis of AIDS, he was able to legally stay. The irony is found in the man's statement 'it is the disease which kills me that has become my reason for living now' (ibid). Biolegitimacy, states Fassin, links the matter of living, the biological, with the meaning of politics. As such, a focus on biolegitimacy rather than biopower 'emphasize[s] the construction of the meaning and values of life instead of the exercise of forces and strategies to control it' (ibid:52). Fassin aims to move the politicised body beyond governmentality and thus move the focus of study 'from the "rules of the game" to its stakes' (ibid). In cases like Surbiton, the stakes are the future of the suburb as a valuable place with a distinct and important character. The stakes are one's own sense of belonging, the sense of place one leaves to the next generation, and – I argue – their health and well-being.

The site that Tim and others were trying to save was intimately tied to their sense of self, the values they held dear, such as ecological and historical value. As such, protection of the site was also a way of protecting themselves and the forms of social relations they wish to enact via the urban landscape. To lose it, they argued, would be to lose part of themselves. As such, the stakes were high. This chapter argues that the practice of performing local citizenship is a necessary act of performing one's biolegitimacy, which must be constantly performed in order to maintain oneself as socially legitimate. In this sense, this chapter is not a discussion of forms of biopower in terms of the way in which human conduct is governed; rather, it is a description of how local citizenship is performed in the processes of a community trying to assert themselves in urban planning procedures. Locals work hard to scale up their personal and local conceptions of the value of the built environment into the processes of urban planning. The chapter outlines how the body and the city are deeply connected and further how, through these emerging practices of being local, of performing one's citizenship, the body somatises the stress and strain of having to maintain a form of biolegitimacy. As such, the body, and the fluids its extrudes, not only give rise to the infrastructures of the city, but also relate to the health effects of being a citizen of the city.

The body and the city

The body and the city have long been linked through metaphor and analogy. Richard Sennett's *Flesh and Stone: The Body and the City in Western Civilisation* (1994) makes the assertion that the urban plans of second-century

Rome were based on idealisations of the body. He traces how the centre is the heart, the parks the lungs, the roads the arteries, and the sewers the guts. The relation between the human mind and the city was evoked in the pioneering urban theory of Lewis Mumford (1938), who stated that cities were a fact of nature, a part of man's natural expression in that the 'mind takes form in the city; and in turn; urban forms condition the mind' (1938:5). More recently, Steve Pile has outlined how the body and the city interact in a complex kind of psychological grid (1996:177) whereby the control, purification, and disciplining of the city is mirrored in the body. Pile draws heavily from historians Stallybrass and White, who describe how

> the reformation of the senses produced, as a necessary corollary, new thresholds of shame, embarrassment and disgust. And in the nineteenth century, those thresholds were articulated above all through specific contents, the slum, the sewer, the nomad, the savage, the rat, which in turn, remapped the body.
>
> (1986:285)

It was, argues Elizabeth Grosz, the rise of scientific rationalism that led to the 'Cartesian split' between the body and the city whereby it comes to be understood that 'humans make cities' (1998:33) with a rational mind which is separate to the body.

By extension, Grosz argues that just as the mind and body have been conceptualised as separate, so too have the body and the city. This subordinates the body to the mind and presumes a one-way relation of the subjectivity of the cause (maker) and the city (the made). For Grosz, this underplays the degree to which the city – in my case, the everyday environment of the suburbs – is a factor in the production of the corporal self. The built environment of the city is a prime organiser of otherwise unrelated bodies. The metaphor of the city as body (see Sennett 1996) serves as justification for forms of 'ideal' government and organisation through a process of naturalisation. The city becomes a parallel of the human body in that it is a natural form of organisation whose functions must be not only for the good of each organ but also primarily for the good of the whole. The parallel between the body and social order saw its clearest formations in the seventeenth century 'when liberal political philosophers justified their various allegiances (the divine right of kings, for Hobbes; parliamentary representation, for Locke; direct representation, for Rousseau, etc.) through the metaphor of the body-politic' (Grosz 1998:33). For Grosz, the question is not simply 'how to distinguish life-enhancing from life-denying environments' but to examine different environments, both in their material politics and their socio-cultural milieu and consider how they 'actively produce the bodies of their inhabitants as particular and distinctive types of bodies, as bodies with particular physiologies, affective lives, and concrete behaviours' (Grosz 1998:35). In this way, I go beyond the theoretical notions of biopower and look at how, through being citizen, a particular form of body, as a manifestation of a political way of being, emerges from being a good 'local.' The 'local' as citizen, that is, a person who involves themselves in the political governance of the city, enacts the body-politic in that they represent the politically responsible demos. The practice of being local is the practice of an inclusive democracy, in this sense, I use the term 'body-politic' (see ahead) to describe a political collective of people but also how the practice of being citizen manifests in an individual's body. But first we must understand why the water filtration site was important to the Surbiton locals, and why Tim would sacrifice and suffer so much to save it.

London's sewers: a recent history of shit

At the turn of the eighteenth century, London's population was around 1 million; one hundred years later, this had swelled to a staggering 6.7 million, making it one of the largest cities in the world at the time. Shit became a problem as Emily Mann reported,

> The steaming hot summer of 1858, the hideous stench of human excrement rising from the River Thames and seeping through the hallowed halls of the Houses of Parliament finally got too much for Britain's politicians – those who had not already fled in fear of their lives to the countryside.
>
> (Mann 2016)

At the time, bad air and 'evil odour' was thought to carry with it the curse of ill health (see Carroll, this volume). Further to the stench, successive epidemics of dysentery, typhoid, and cholera saw pressure mount for solutions to the great stink. The outcome has been described as 'one of history's most life-enhancing advancements in urban planning' which 'laid the foundation for modern London' (Mann 2016). The solution was Joseph Bazalgette's sewage system composed of 82 miles of new sewers and subterranean boulevards, which is still the basis of London's sewage system today. This will be updated in 2023 with a 'super sewer' built, according to Peter Ackroyd, 'in the spirit of Bazalgette' (Mann 2016). Before Bazalgette's sewer, London, as it is understood today, was divided into different administrations. The Old City, The Metropolitan Regions, and the Square Mile all had different city commissioners, infrastructural plans, and approaches (if any at all) to managing waste, people, buildings, and so on. The Poor Law Commissioner, Edwin Chadwick, urged the different administrations to clean up their territories; however, it was not until 1848 that the City Sewers Act saw widespread infrastructural development of water systems and Bazalgette, as chief engineer of the Metropolitan Board of Works, began work on the sewers. Chadwick, however, was still a follower of the miasmic theory, believing that cholera was passed through bad air, and as such cholera was not linked to water supply. The 'great experiment' of Dr John Snow proved that cholera was, in fact, transmitted through infected water. Snow contrasted the health of people who drew water from the Lambeth Water Company with that of those who drew from Southwark and Vauxhall who drew water from the Thames at Battersea. Inspired by Francis Bacon and the scientific method, Snow aligned two populations, Lambeth water drinkers and Southwark and Vauxhall water drinkers, with all other variables the same to see if there was a difference in incidence. This 'grand experiment' was interrupted by another epidemic, and Snow, a practicing GP based in SoHo, saw many incidences of cholera. Snow famously traced these local cases to the Broad Street pump. This pump, upon excavation, was shown to contain faeces which had leaked from a neighbouring cesspit. Snow's proof was only due to his ability to trace and map clean water. Snow traced clean water back to its sources, one of which emerged from James Simpson's new water filtration systems in Surbiton (Seething Wells Water 2013).

These water filtration beds used a new method of filtering which purified the water by removing floating particles and dirt. Until the mid-1800s, dirty water had been desirable and was seen to hold life-giving properties. However, with development in medical science, the microscope and understandings of health and disease, clear water was now desired. Not only did these filtration systems clean the water but also, unexpectedly, the settling process allowed bacteria to form on the surface of the water, which actively removed cholera. This filtration system, the understanding of health and disease, and the associated engineering projects are still the basis of London's sewer and clean water systems and have influenced the management of clean water and excrement around the world. It was these filtration beds that led people to change their desire from opaque water to clear water. The dirt had become just that, 'matter out of place' (Douglas 1966:1). Surbiton's filter beds were fundamental in the story of clean water, the rise of modern epidemiology, the abjection of shit, and the history of urban planning. Before these developments, shit was not as abject and rejected as it became.

The historical contingency of shit

In the book *The History of Shit* (2000) Dominique Laporte outlines a historical genealogy of shit and draws on Foucault, Freud, and Descartes, amongst others, to show how the development of sanitation techniques in Europe affected notions of modern self. For Laporte, the removal of shit to the private realm was synonymous with the founding of the modern family and bourgeois subjectivity. Laporte argues that 'until the very eve of clinical medicine, it was maintained that shit had the potential to be unquestionably good' owing to its fertile qualities. However, the rise of the private family unit and individual sense of self (following Freud and Mill) or, as Laporte states, 'the Cartesian ideology of the I' (ibid:32), saw shit and its cesspools washed away and relegated to the private realm. Laporte argues that shit was not 'pernicious in and of itself . . . only through its recent association with the body' keeping as it did the body's legacy of original sin (ibid:36). Shit, then, must be collected, and is done in huge volumes, by the state. Laporte argues that this produces a binding dialectic between the state and the individual:

> Totalitarianism speaks thus: Methodically collect your manure and give it to the State that wishes you well. Give up this shit, this fruit of your labour, and in return, I will fulfil all your needs and lavish you with such gifts that you shall lack for nothing.
>
> (ibid:129)

For Laporte, the history of the utilitarian relation to the management of shit and the physiological movements of the body can be understood only within the context of the prevailing social attitudes to our bodies. The effects of this bodily relation and the private position of shit, which is to be neither smelt nor seen outside the confines of the home, are also to be seen in the construction of the built environment, not just in the sewer systems but also in domestic furnishing, streets, public squares, and the urban public realm.

Rabinow (1989) traces how the 'social' and the modern form of 'society' emerged in France along with new forms of government that was seen to be justified and needed in order to deal with the cholera epidemic. Rabinow, working with Foucault's notion of 'biopower,' which relates to 'an explosion of numerous and diverse techniques for achieving the subjugation of bodies and the control of populations' (Foucault 1978:141), argued that a particular modern relation of the individual to the state came about through this constellation of city, state, and the management of fluids. These developments are today seen as the 'foundation' of our modern cities and in many ways the foundation of the modern, urban, subjectivity. In 2007, the United Nations Population Fund predicted that in the following year over half the world population would be living in cities (NFPA 2007). However, Vaughan et al. (2009) note that in Europe and North America, at least, most residents of cities (84%) are actually living in the suburbs, which have, even since the times of Mumford, always been considered a little abject.

The suburbs: a bit shit?

Surbiton, home of Simpson's water filter beds, has a reputation as the queen of the suburbs, it even sounds like suburb: 'Suburbiton' (*London Evening Standard* 2012; *The Big Issue* 1999). In 1995, Liverpool City Council 'seriously considered adopting "Liverpool – it's not Surbiton" as a marketing slogan' (Statham 1996: xiii in Wickstead 2013). In 1999, *The Big Issue* magazine ran an editorial feature, 'I Want the Good Life,' with the subtitle

'Bland. Boring. Banal. Everything You Think You Know about Suburbia is Wrong; says Jim McClellan and to prove it, he's moving to Surbiton.' The magazine professed to be surprised that there was actually 'life' in the suburbs. Railing against this reputation the residents of Surbiton have been particularly active at fostering their own sense of community. They regularly hold events and festivals in order to get people together and have fun. A Community Interest Company (CIC), 'The Community Brain,' was established in the area in order to foster such community spirit. A CIC is a company whose primary purpose is the community and uses business solutions and structure to deliver public good, often run by volunteers as a non-profit. CICs have emerged since 2005 under the 2004 'Audit, Investigations and Community Enterprise Act.' The encouragement of this form of community organising ran parallel with the localism agenda of central government to devolve political power to local authorities and local people, manifest in the 2011 Localism Act. The Community Brain aimed to foster a sense of community, stating on its website that its objectives are

> to carry on activities which benefit the community in particular anyone who believes they are outside of a perceived, meaningful community. This could be people isolated by culture, geography, poverty, disability or simply a lack of connection with the people around them.
>
> (The Community Brain 2013)

For The Community Brain, it was important that people get together regardless of political differences and viewpoints: the idea was to foster familiarity and trust with each other and develop community. Steve, a prominent community leader and organiser, described to me how one day he was walking by the old water filtration site and he started to wonder about the place in more detail. The site had not been used since the mid-1970s and is largely hidden from everyday view, owing to its sunken location behind a brick wall wedged between a busy road. Steve visited the local history archives and was astonished at the site's links to the story of cholera and clean water. He explained how for 20 years he had

> *walked past some lovely blue railings by the side of the road and never paid them any attention. . . . I never really took the time, stopped to look, or paid attention to the site . . . allowed it to come into focus, . . . we've got something on our doorstep here.*

In 2013, the community carried out extensive research on the site with the help of a Community Heritage Grant that brought stories of the site 'to life.' Increasing numbers of people in the local community came to understand the site through its history, its place in the story of modern epidemiology, clean water, and city building and through the potentials of unique urban ecology through presentations, talks, and community gossip. A play,

'The story of King Cholera,' was held in a disused pump house, delivering a rich history to the community from within the site. The site's ecological importance, which has developed since its retirement as a water filtration site, means that it is one of the few areas of open still water in London. As such, a rare bat species, the Daubenton, feeds over the site and a web blog sees the anthropomorphised 'Benton the Bat'[1] answer questions about his ecology from a website that tracks the wildlife on the site. Benton has also been made into a puppet and parades around the local area during community events whilst leaflets about his life are handed out. Such events allow affiliation and familiarity with the site's histories and ecologies. Through such events, the site became vibrant and grew in popularity and importance as the local community invested in it emotionally and physically. The site's importance to the local community grew as the stories of its history and the unique ecologies, in the words of Tim, threatened to 'put Surbiton on the map.'

At the same time as the community learned about the site through the heritage grant, Lake Properties, who had bought the land, submitted a planning application to build luxury homes. The community quickly formed the Friends of Seething Wells Association (FoSWA), a CIC that would spearhead the opposition to Lake's plans. Tim, a key researcher on the community project, took the lead role in FoSWA. This involved organising meetings, keeping records, setting up a special business bank account for the CIC, fundraising, involving a wider public, getting local MPs on side, courting press, and setting up and maintaining websites. Tim was by no means alone, but the work was significant, and Tim was a pivotal figurehead for the group. Eventually, at the council planning meeting, Tim was to give five minutes of evidence on behalf of the community on why the application should be refused. FoSWA was given permission to speak on their basis of being a CIC, a recognised local interest group.

The body politic

On the night of the meeting, I caught Steve waiting nervously outside the main hall as he moved from person to person, thanking them for coming as they entered the room. With a smile and hug, I asked how he was feeling. 'Sick,' he replied with a sharp and serious demeanour before walking off to greet someone else with a smile. Throughout the meeting, Steve, wearing a black shirt, stood by the door, bit his nails, and even cried a little. Steve suffers from bi-polar depression and wears a black shirt when unwell and white shirt whilst well. His does this so that those who know him may be able to be aware and offer support. He had been wearing a black shirt for months before the meeting decision and told me that the whole process had

---

1 Benton has his own website, Accessed 12 January 2018. http://bentonbat.blogspot.co.uk/.

made him very unwell. Steve felt viscerally responsible for ensuring the filter beds where protected, that local people supported the objection and could see the objection as a form of protection for the future. Steve had told an audience at a public meeting some weeks before that he worried that if these filter beds and their histories were lost, future generations might ask 'where were you?' For Steve, protection of the beds was also protection of particular values, ecologies, and histories, a protection of a source of local pride to be passed on to the next generation.

Tim was supported at the meeting by Benny, who also gave evidence. Benny was a professional heritage expert who lived in the area. He was the lead investigator on the community Lottery-funded heritage project that initially animated the site with the history of cholera. Some months before the council meeting, Benny and I finished leading a heritage walk around the perimeter of the filter beds before moving to the pub for a quiet drink. We overlooked a sunset shimmering off the filter beds as Benny explained to me how he had been careful not to get too involved in FoSWA. He felt he had to distance himself from the whole objection process for his own good, describing in viscerally corporal terms:

BENNY: *It's a funny one . . . I just had to move away from it all really, I just don't know, you know, I don't know what I would do if it doesn't work.*
ME: *What? If they win?*
BENNY: *Yeah . . ., if Lake win, I'm not sure what I'll do, I'm not sure I can take that, I'm so involved, too much, it would tear me apart to be honest, I've got so much of me in there, to see it just built on and all that lost, I'm not sure I could take it to be honest. I have to be careful; I'm trying not to give too much of myself.*

Benny talked in direct corporal terms about being 'torn apart' and having 'so much of me in there,' but referring to the effect of being a good local citizen through the body is more than mere analogy. Steve told me of the direct effects on his health; this was something that Tim was also to make clear later.

In the months leading up the planning meeting, I saw less and less of Tim. I had built a close personal relationship with Tim through my ethnography of the community events and helping with Heritage tours. Meetings, interviews, and hanging out with Tim were becoming rarer as he increasingly cancelled, rearranged, or was less present at these events. Months after the council decision, Tim explained how he had been through an incredibly hard time. His wife did not approve of him spending large amounts of time away from the home. His marriage was breaking down, and he had grown distant from his son. Tim explained that he felt he had developed an unhealthy relationship to alcohol, particularly as community meetings were invariably held in pubs and to stay for a pint was something that was hugely socially productive, as it 'eased tensions and built bonds.' Reflecting on the objection process, I told Tim that, to me, he appeared calm and controlled, rational and collected during the council meeting itself. Tim then declared that he actually he was sweating profusely throughout the meeting and that in the months before and after the meeting, his stress had manifested in irritable bowels or, as he put it, 'deep in my guts.' During the council meeting, he explained, he was distracted by needing multiple visits to the bathroom. He told me that on one occasion, he was 'shitting profusely' and that he 'felt dizzy and almost blacked out. . . . I thought I was having a stroke.' Whilst Tim was clearly proud of his achievements and the appreciation the community had shown him for his significant efforts, in this moment of quiet reflection over a drink, he told me some of the negative aspects of the process. It had taken a long time for Tim to talk about this with me, and he admitted that he had not really talked to anyone about it. He apologised for the cancelled meetings but explained that he did not really want 'the anthropologist,' one who may go on to represent the more positive aspects of community events, to see him struggling. Tim was clearly trying to present a vision of community that 'worked' and citizens which 'work.' He stated that he did not want to moan or appear to complain, and that if the objection happened again, which it was threatening to do through an appeal process, he would do it all again. As such, these sufferings seem to be the necessary aspect of being a citizen. Tim explained it in such terms: 'I saw protecting the filter beds as looking after the child of tomorrow,' but for Tim, that meant 'I didn't look after the child of today [referring to his son] quite as I would like.'

Returning to the declaration that I had witnessed 'a community that worked,' I consider 'work' in two ways. First, the local residents had been successful in thwarting a planning application to build on a site of community interest. Second, this success was the result of much hard labour in the form of organising meetings, gaining local support, and working through tiresome bureaucratic processes. The consequence of this 'work,' understood as a moral necessity in an age marked by ideals of inclusion, participation, and localism in democracy, is manifest not only in the preservation of a particular site of community interest, but also in the subjectivities and dispositions of the people involved. The 'local' citizens felt the bodily effect of democratic participation through depression, anxiety, and irritable bowels, the seemingly worthwhile price of 'a community that works.'

The irony of inclusion

It seems that we have come full circle. The problem of managing the abject substance of shit as it emerged, alongside the rise of scientific rationalism and increased understanding of health and disease, as a health-threatening, foul-smelling substance, gave rise to the particular infrastructures and forms of governance that mark the modern city and urban citizenship today. Shit was managed for the benefit of the health of the population and such infrastructures, scientific achievements, and technical advances became part of the narrative of the city, embedded in the materiality of the landscape and source of local pride for residents who felt infrastructure such as the filter beds tied them to bigger stories of the city. Ironically, this pride led to the community having to defend the site from development. This action resulted in Tim, and others, undergoing a huge amount of stress that manifested in ill health and gave rise to unruly shit.

I argue that this ill health is deeply ironic (see Lambek and Antze 2003). Nehamas states that 'irony is acknowledged concealment' (1998:67); 'irony allows you simply to let your audience know what you think and to suggest simply that it is not what you say' (ibid:55). 'Irony,' he continues later,

> allows us to pretend we are something other than our words suggest. It enables us to play at being someone, without forcing us to decide what we really are or, indeed, whether we really are anyone. . . . Irony always and necessarily postulates a double speaker and a double audience.
>
> (ibid:59–60)

In this sense, Tim's shit was embodied irony in that while he was attempting to be a good citizen, to celebrate and protect the narrative of epidemiology and the management of shit, as manifest in the materiality of the suburb, this very attempt gave him unruly shit. Tim's doublespeak was the outward presentation of the good local citizen and the inward manifestation of the stress this produced. This double bind (cf. Bateson et al. 1956) is the condition of being a good local in a landscape where the political impetus to protect a site's local value against an otherwise inevitable market force, the building of luxury flats, lies with the local citizen. This 'de-statization' of governance demands that local people, local communities take on the responsibility of their own maintenance as legitimate, valued forms of life through the performance of citizenship.

In this sense, Tim and the other locals were performing what Ilana Gershon might call 'neoliberal agency' (Gershon 2011). Gershon outlines how the neoliberal subject possess a reflexive kind of agency whereby the self is conceived as a flexible bundle of skills which is able to be managed as though a business in order to best navigate neoliberal landscapes of risk. Gershon focuses particularly on individuals who sculpt a presentation of themselves as flexible and adaptable in responsive to the market demands for flexible workers. However, in my case, locals have used community events and organising to develop what they call a 'resilient community.' They have cultivated the skills, resources, and energy of the community in order to be able to cohere an organised and strategic response to a planning application. They were able to manage the risk that the application posed to the site, which by extension was a threat to themselves and their sense of local pride and their sense of the future. I argue that the time and energy of locals to socially organise and protect those aspects of themselves they saw deeply tied to the filter beds resulted in not only particular local socialities but also particular bodies.

In this sense, the position of the suburban local is one of deep irony whereby they are in a double bind. They are not excluded from the political life of the city, rather they are invited to come and be the very substance of the body politic, the demos of democracy. It is through performing their citizenship that they are able to sculpt the city and maintain the material qualities of the built environment. However, the very practice of doing so has very real and tangible health effects. Shit is at the heart of this; it is the unruly substance that needed to be managed. The management of shit gave rise to modern infrastructures and forms of governance and citizenship that demark the modern city and the sense of self of a city subject. However, the frame of neoliberal market logics remains strong and as such, the position of a 'community that works' is that of a community that is both successful but also one that labours. This labour has its effects in the tension manifest in the gut and extruded, in an unruly manner, as shit.

Conclusion

This chapter has outlined how the practice of being a good local, through partaking in local politics and objecting to a planning application, enables the moral and political position of citizenship in liberal democracies to be enacted. This position, however, takes work to protect those aspects of the materiality of the built environment which have come to be considered an aspect of the local self, such as the filter beds, which results in ill health. This chapter highlights particular aspects of the bodily condition that emerge from such work. The irony, of course, is that the very condition of developing unruly shit emerged from the effort to protect an infrastructure that was constructed to manage shit. Just as shit become abject with the rise of scientific rationalism, so the shit of modern citizenship is often hidden as part of being citizen. It is considered a failed aspect of managing the self in relation to the citizen position, an unhappy and unsuccessful aside to the success of a community that works. This chapter has shown how that materiality of the city is deeply tied to the materiality of the body. One does not emerge from the other, nor is the city merely symbolic of the body but rather both the form of urban materialities and bodily materialities are in a binding dialectic. They can be understood only in this particular moment as coming about together and as such bodies that live in cities should be considered with and through the city itself. Extending this assertion, one could ask how housing or transport infrastructure effects health through stressful commutes, air pollution, or strain on finances. The city is more than a metaphor for the body, and it is more than a material manifestation of the mind. Rather, the city is the material through which the politics of being included in the demos, the politics of the city, a politically qualified social life, is played out. In this sense, the practice of being a citizen requires work; labour which results both in a successful legitimatisation of one's lifeform but also in stress somatising in the guts and affected the very form of bodily of experience an urban citizen has. In this sense, citizenship comes at a cost; sometimes that cost is shit.

References

Bateson, G., D. D. Jackson, J. Haley, and J. Weakland (1956). Toward a theory of schizophrenia. *Systems Research and Behavioral Science* 1(4):251–264.

The Community Brain, Website. Accessed 12 January 2013. http://thecommunity brain.org/

Douglas, M. P. (1966). *Purity and Danger: An Analysis of Concepts of Pollution and Taboo*. London: Routledge.

Fassin, D. (2009). Another politics of life is possible. *Theory, Culture & Society* 26(5):44–60.

Foucault, M. (1978). *The History of Sexuality: The Will to Knowledge (Vol 1)*. Trans R. Hurley. London: Penguin Books.

Gershon, I. (2011). Neoliberal agency. *Current Anthropology* 52(4):537–555.

Grosz, E. (1998). Bodies-cities. In H. Nast and S. Pile (Eds.), *Places Through The Body*. London and New York: Routledge.

I Want the Good Life. (1999). *The Big Issue Magazine*, 16–17.

Lambek, M., and P. Antze (Eds.) (2003). *Illness and Irony: On the Ambiguity of Suffering in Culture*. New York. Berghahn Books.

Laporte, D. (2000). *History of Shit*. Cambridge, MA: MIT Press.

Lewis, M. (1938). *The Culture of Cities*. New York: Harcourt, Brace and Co.

Mann, E. (2016). Story of cities #14: London's Great Stink heralds a wonder of the industrial world. *The Guardian*. Accessed 4 April 2016. www.theguardian.com/cities/2016/apr/04/story-cities-14-london-great-stink-river-thames-joseph-bazalgette-sewage-system.

Mumford, L., (1938). *The Culture of Cities*. New York: Harcourt, Brace and Co.

Nehamas, A. (1998). *The art of Living: Socratic Reflections from Plato to Foucault (Vol. 61)*. California: University of California Press.

Pile, S. (1996). *The Body and the City: Psychoanalysis, Space and Subjectivity*. London and New York: Routledge.

Rabinow, P. (1989). *French Modern: Norms and Forms of the Social Environment*. Chicago: University of Chicago Press.

Rose, N. (1996). Governing "Advanced" Liberal Democracies. In A. Barry, T. Osborne and N. Rose (Eds.), *Foucault and Political Reason: Liberalism, Neo-liberalism and Rationalities of Government*. Chicago: University of Chicago Press, 37–64.

Seething Wells (2013). Water – Surbiton's Hidden Heritage. Public Blog. Accessed 3 April 2014. http://seethingwellswater.org/Seething_Wells_-_Surbitons_Hidden_Heritage.html.

Sennett, R. (1996). *Flesh and Stone: The Body and the City in Western Civilization*. WW Norton & Company.

Sharma, A., and A. Gupta (2006). The anthropology of the state: A reader. *Blackwell Readers in Anthropology* 13:9.

Stallybrass, P., and A. White (1986). *The Politics and Poetics of Transgression*. London: Methuen, 125–148.

Statham, R. (1996). *Surbiton Post*. Phillimore: Guildford, Surrey.

Vaughan, L., S. Griffiths, M. Haklay and C.E. Jones (2009). Do the suburbs exist? Discovering complexity and specificity in suburban built form. *Transactions of the Institute of British Geographers* 34(4):475–488.

Wickstead, H. (2013). The Goat Boy of Mount Seething: Heritage and the English Suburbs. In M. Dines and T. Vermeulen (Eds.), *New Suburban Stories*. London and New York: Continuum, 199–213.

12 Of smoke and unguents
Health affordances of sacred materiality

Timothy Carroll

Introduction

This chapter asks, what is the affordance of the person and its substances such that materials can be scripted within the health and maintenance of its being? It begins with a historic investigation of how the burning of incense was understood and practiced (or avoided) in the first five centuries of the Christian faith. Looking at Patristic sources (i.e. the writing of the Church fathers) as well as subsequent scholarship concerning ancient medicinal and ritual uses of incense, the chapter seeks to trace the lines of interconnection between the resins, their properties, affordances, and uses, as well as the ways the materials were understood to impact the person. The chapter then turns to contemporary liturgical practice within the Orthodox Christian Church. In this context, some similar motifs still exist; however, the particulars of why and how materials impact upon the person have changed. I conclude the chapter exploring the implications for how health and the person are understood in relation to the substances of medicinal use.

Methodologically, I am reading the ancient sources as an ethnographer, not as a historiographer. While aware of some of the historical and historiographical debates about antiquity and the textual traditions upon which I am drawing, I am more concerned with how the writers – as ethnographic informants – express their world.[1] As such, the historical section of this chapter includes some long quotations, chosen in part to provide a sense of the voice from this earlier period.

Historical context

Mediterranean religion in antiquity was rich with olfaction. This was true across the Greco-Roman forms of paganism as well as temple Judaism.

---

1 I find some justification in reading these ancient sources as ethnographies in following Stephen Tyler's (1987) argument that the original ethnography was the Bible. While the authors I am citing are not those found in the Scriptures, they would have seen themselves in the same genre and intertextual tradition that produced the Bible.

Everybody used incense, and a wide variety of substances – mostly plants, oils, and spices – were burned in ritual contexts. Some, such as storax (a somewhat vague category, including resins from various plants in the Altingiaceae and Styracaceae families) grew natively, but many of the more highly desired were imported at great cost from Arabia, Africa, or India. For my purpose, here, I am most interested in frankincense *(Boswellia sacra)*. The material could be mixed and administered in a number of media, and it 'was used in fumigation, salve, potions and pills. It was also part of some oil-based perfumes and unguents. Medicines, efficient in liquid forms, also could be burnt as incense' (Caseau 2007:79). The historical record does not always specify what kind of resin was being used, and along with storax and frankincense, myrrh *(Commiphora myrrha)* was (and is) also common. Where the historical record tends to be more specific is not in the ritual context, but in the medical context. Here, in the writings of, for example, Pedanius Dioscorides (c. 40–90 CE) and Galen of Pergamon (c. 129–210 CE), frankincense and other tree resins are medical substances with clearly delineated properties and applications. In his five-volume *De Materia Medica*, Dioscorides outlines various ways of processing frankincense, called *'thus'* in this context, and outlines its medical applications, saying:

> It is able to warm and is an astringent to clean away things which darken the pupils, fill up the hollowness of ulcers and draw them to a scar, and to glue together bloody wounds; and it is able to suppress all excessive discharges of blood including that of the neural membrane. Pounded into small pieces and applied with linen dipped in milk it lessens malignant ulcers around the perineum and other parts. . . . It is effective mixed with medicines made for the arteries and the bowels; and taken as a drink it helps those who spit blood. . . . *Thus* is burnt in a clean ceramic jar and set on fire by a piece of it lighted by a candle until it is burnt. You must (after it is fully burnt) stop it with something until it is quenched, for so it will not be turned into ashes. Some also put a hollow brass jar around the pot with holes in the middle for receiving the soot, as we will show in the description of the soot of *thus*. Some place it into unfired jars, wrap it around with clay, and burn it in a furnace. It is also burnt in a new ceramic jar with hot burning coals until it no longer bubbles nor sends out any more fat or vapour, and that which is thoroughly burnt is easily broken.
>
> (2000:85–86)

The soot gained by gathering the smoke rising from burned *thus*, like that rising from burned myrrh and storax (2000:88) was known, Dioscorides tells us, to have 'the ability to soothe inflammation of the eyes, repress discharges, clean ulcers, fill hollow sores, and repress diseases of the cornea' (2000:87). In later Eastern Roman medicine, frankincense continued to be used due to its antiseptic qualities, wherein after surgery to remove a kidney stone the wound was filled with manna [a paste made of frankincense] and clean, warm wool impregnated with olive oil and then bandaged. The dressing was changed two or three times a day and once at night, and the wound was washed with copious olive oil. After the third day, healing medicines were applied to the incision until new flesh appeared. Then a plaster with vinegar and oil was applied until healing was complete.

(Lascaratos et al. 2004:806)

The rheumic and antiseptic qualities of frankincense worked both as manna and when incinerated. The burning of incense, then, was good for the eyes, lungs, and skin, amongst other things.

It is also worth noting, that in some cases, the burning of incense in Mediterranean antiquity was not clearly delineated as either ritual or medicinal. They were not mutually exclusive domains. Hippocrates had taught that all disease was airborne, and while Dioscorides and Galen after him both rejected the exclusivity of the statement, the predominant understanding that disease was at least principally airborne carried on. As such, foul smells took on a dangerous aspect, and they were replaced by equally aerially mobile good, agreeable scents (Caseau 2007:77–78). Even when discussing ritualised incense use within a temple complex, the use may be best understood as principally medicinal, as can be seen, for example, in the censing of the Isiac temple each evening, not as a sacrifice to Isis, but so as to clean the air for the health of the resident priests. Writing of this Egyptian practice, Plutarch (46–125 CE) notes that 'the element of health is no less important than that of piety' (Plutarch 1936:185; cf. Caseau 2007:79).

Into this milieu, the first generations of Christians struggled to articulate their difference. Authors like Justin Martyr (c. 160 CE) argued that 'God has no need of streams of blood, libations, and incense' (Justin Martyr 1885:166), emphasising that the sacrificial economy of Christianity was distinct from that of both the pagans and the Jews. Nonetheless, the imagery of incense and sacrifice was still pervasive and seen to be persuasive. The martyrdom account of Polycarp (c. 155 CE) records that after refusing to make a sacrifice to the Roman gods, and to swear the oath to the greatness of Caesar, the bishop of Smyrna was condemned to die at the stake. Those who witnessed his death attested to the final sequence of his passion as follows:

A great flame blazed up and those of us to whom it was given to see beheld a miracle. And we have been preserved to recount the story to others. For the flames, bellying out like a ship's sail in the wind, formed into the shape of a vault and thus surrounded the martyr's body as with a wall. And he was within it not as burned flesh but rather as bread being baked, or like gold and silver being purified in a smelting furnace. And from it we perceived such a delightful fragrance as though it were smoking incense or some other costly perfume. At last when the vicious men realised that his body could not be consumed by the fire they ordered a confector [executioner] to go up and plunge a dagger

into the body. When he did this there came out such a quantity of blood
that the flames were extinguished.

(quoted in Ashbrook Harvey 2006:12)

Along with the various parallels with Christ's own sacrifice – such as the
gushing of liquid coming forth after being stabbed – and earlier Jewish
martyrology – such as the three youths in the Babylonian furnace – there is
also a new set of martyric tropes emerging. The bread, for one, is an important symbol of the Christian faith, linking the sacrifice of Polycarp to the
preparation of the loaf that would be used in the Eucharistic feast and other
communal acts of benefaction.[2] Fresh bread was (and is) an integral part
of Christian gatherings, and an olfactory link between the smell of baking
bread and the liturgical sacrifice of the Eucharist would be a salient image
to those reading Polycarp's martyrography. Developing the olfactory scene
of the martyrdom, however, the authors attest to the scent of frankincense.[3]
This starts a long and ornate tradition of the smell of frankincense and/or
myrrh (often as sweet rose, or sometimes as sweet basil) being present at a
martyrdom or at the discovery of relics.[4]

The link between the sacred and fragrance was pervasive in late antiquity,
and on this point, Christians agreed with their counterparts. God Himself
was understood as 'perfect fragrance' (Athenagoras 1885:134), and the fragrance of Old Testament sacrificial offering was interpreted to have moral
implications (see, for example, Chrysostom 1979:27). The resistance to
incense, particularly strong in the Latin West, related to the use of incense
as a sacrifice before the Roman gods as the minimal obligation of political
allegiance (Brent 2010:182). In this political climate, the ritual burning of
incense took on an association with the denial of Christ and the murder of
thousands of Christians who refused to burn incense in this context.

Throughout this entire period, however, it is important to note that,
even within the Latin context where the Christian rejection of incense is
most vocal, it is only the ritual use of it that gains Patristic ire. Tertullian
(c. 155–220 CE), one of the most loquacious in his aversion to incense and
perfumes, admits that there is nothing inherently wrong with the substances
themselves (Ashbrook Harvey 2006:36). As he says,

> The substances [used in sacrifice and libation] are themselves as creatures
> of God without impurity, and in this their native state are free to the use

---

2 Maybe worth noting the importance of bread in early Christian theology, in such concepts
of 'one bread' (1 Corinthians 10.17) which Christians partake of in the Eucharist. There are
also obvious links with Jewish antecedents which link bread with blessing.

3 Ashbrook Harvey simply says 'smoking incense,' whereas the same line appears in the Ante-
Nicene Fathers series as 'we perceived such a sweet odour [coming from the pile], as if frankincense or some such precious spices had been smoking [literally 'breathing'] there' (Coxe
1885:42).

4 See, as one classic example, various accounts of the Empress Helena finding the True Cross
in Jerusalem, in 326 CE (cf. Ashbrook Harvey 2006:65).

of all; but the ministries to which in their use they are devoted, makes all the difference; for I, too, kill a cock for myself, just as Socrates did for Æsculapius; and if the smell of some place or other offends me, I burn the Arabian product myself, but not with the same ceremony, nor in the same dress, nor with the same pomp, with which it is done to idols.

(Tertullian 1885:99)

Clement of Alexandria (c. 150–215 CE) too balances his warning against perfumes, flowers, oils, and incense with scientific knowledge of the time concerning the health benefits of olfactory regiments. After admitting the 'individual properties, some beneficial, some injurious, some also dangerous' of various plants, he summarises, saying, 'We have showed that in the department of medicine, for healing, and sometimes also for moderate recreation, the delight derived from flowers, and the benefit derived from ointments and perfumes, are not to be overlooked' (Clement 1885:257; see also Caseau 2007:78).

In this context, it was common for incense to be burned in the home and in public buildings. It was good for one's health. As a form of preventative medicine, it cleaned the air against disease, drove away vermin such as mice and snakes, and also served as prescribed medication against various ailments. It was also commonly burned in tombs, catacombs, and wakes. It drove away the stench and freshened and purified the air. While Christians rejected the ritual use of incense as a sacrifice, they accept the scientific and medical knowledge about it and maintained the cultural uses for it.

Christian liturgical use of incense

The fourth century saw a marked shift in the acceptance of incense in the Church. The legalisation of the religion (313 CE) meant that Christian subjects of Rome were no longer required to participate in incense sacrifices to the gods and the emperor. Another factor, however, is that Constantine's reign, and particularly his mother's investment in the Levant, saw an increase in the importance of the cultural practices in the eastern reaches of the empire. The Church in Syria and Jerusalem never expressed as strong a resistance against the use of incense as its Latin counterparts did. It should not be a surprise, then, that the first certain usage of incense in Christian liturgical practice is witnessed by the pilgrim Etheria (or Egeria) in Jerusalem (c. 381), where the tomb of the Holy Sepulchre (within which the body of Christ is reputed to have been laid) is censed midway through the liturgy.

With this first eyewitness account, it is hard to know exactly why incense was used, and it is debated within classicist and historiographical context. It is suggested that Etheria witnessed something like a pageantry of Christ's funeral, re-enacted within the space of his burial (Gero 1977:75), possibly with specific connection to the role of the myrrh-bearing women who, in the Gospel account, carried myrrh and costly spices to anoint Christ's body (Ashbrook Harvey 2006:77). In this interpretation, the use of incense is a play-act in celebration of the death of Christ and the subsequent emptiness of the tomb. This would have fit within Christian practices around death, which, as Tertullian pointed out, included as much incense 'in the burying of Christians as [the pagans use] in the fumigating of the gods' (1885:49). Jerusalem (and, specifically, the Holy Sepulchre) was, however, an example of how the pageantry of liturgy and pilgrimage should be done elsewhere, and it fits with art historical evidence (Hahn 1997) that, even if it was not used in this way at the time, seeing incense used in the liturgy in Jerusalem, the practice would spread further afield.

The other historically contested account linking incense within a Christian place of worship is the *Liber Pontificalis Ecclesiae Romanae* in which it is recorded that Constantine, along with founding the first Roman basilicas, gifted the basilicas quite a significant amount of incense and nard, along with the lamps and censors in which to burn them. Instructions are included, suggesting that the censors were placed in front of the altar. I am largely uninterested in the contested nature of the documents themselves, as Béatrice Caseau (2007:90–91) points out, the documents extant are too erratic – detailed in some places, oddly abridged in others – to suggest a forgery; it seems more likely that the extant copies are the work of lazy, but not inventive, copyists. Nonetheless, it is odd to think that – only shortly after the Edict of Milan put an end to Christian persecution – the emperor would gift the Church something associated with martyrdom and idolatry. Two options exist, however. The first is that burning incense in such a public space could have been for the general health of priests and others using the space – purifying the air as in other situations. The second is that Constantine, in setting up incense burning in front of the altar of the Christian God, would be giving to God the honour previously due to himself, as emperor.

Whatever Constantine's motives, there is a marked shift in Christian attitude towards incense. References in the mid- to late fourth century are often ambiguous and unclear as to if the incense spoken of is literal, metaphorical (as prayer), or both (Ashbrook Harvey 2006; Gero 1977). Within this shift, a major influence in setting the tone for subsequent understanding is Ephrem the Syrian (306–373), whose hymnography is still sung today in the Orthodox churches. He lived during this turning point in Christian attitudes towards incense and having never experienced the negative association between incense and paganism, filled his writing with rich metaphor and theological implication. In his hymns, eating and smelling are similar experiences (even as they are recognised to be in neuroscience), and both bring the Christian into tangible bodily experience of Christ who is both the Fragrance and Bread of Life. In communion, and by inhaling the sweet fragrance, Christ penetrates the Christian:

> Through the act of breathing – the life force itself – Christ's presence saturates the believer. Interestingly, it is fragrance rather than breath that Ephrem highlights again and again; his olfactory imagery is about encounter, not animation. The breath of life that Adam received at

creation animated his lifeless body. The fragrance of Christ inhaled by the believer indicates by its smell the action of human/divine encounter through sensory experience.

(Ashbrook Harvey 2006:113)

Ephrem holds onto the traditions laid down before him, in terms of God (and, specifically, Christ, in most of Ephrem's work) as being pure fragrance, specifically the 'Fragrance of Life,' but develops it in terms of how the material substance of the incense and perfume entangle the body, permeate it, and become united to/within it. His play with the images of fragrance and breath also moves forward the medical ideas about incense and pure air into a conception of the incense as purificatory for the soul. Christ, as perfume, permeates the person body and soul, and even as the breath of life animated the lifeless body of Adam in the Genesis account of creation, so too did the inhalation of the fragrance of Christ bring (new) life and regeneration into the Christian: 'The fragrance of Christ inhaled by the believer indicated by its smell the action of human-divine encounter through sensory experience' (2006:64). This bodily relationship to Christ via the penetrative capacity of incense shapes contemporary perspectives on incense use and prayer.

By the end of the fifth century, Christian practice regularly used incense, in both public and private devotion, and by the sixth century, incense is specifically sought out in order to make supplicatory prayer (Ashbrook Harvey 2006; Atchley 1909). Incense became synecdochic for the larger framework of prayer and the relationship of mediation and fellowship between the human and the divine. With the collapse of paganism, the use of incense also came to be used as an offering given to God or a saint, accompanying prayer for healing or forgiveness (Caseau 2007:92). It also took on a prophylactic quality and was seen to be a demonifuge (2007:84).

An important distinction was made between the fragrance and the substance holding the fragrance. The incense, for its part, was an offering from human kind. Oil was a protective substance, given by the divine to mankind for her well-being – both health and safety. The fragrance itself, however, was divine. The scent of God was the somatic evidence of God's presence. The interplay of substances and odours, then, fit within the cultural and theological understandings of human-divine interaction. The affordance of oil, to coat the skin, and then fuse into it, gives a period of transformation when the flesh of the body is visibly transfigured – made resplendent with the luminescence of the unguent. The pungent aroma, however, instantaneously transfuses the membrane of the body and is there: flush in the nostrils and lungs of the supplicant.

Contemporary use

Today, incense is an integral component of the olfactory, visual, and – because bells are often hung from the chains of censors – aural experience of

Orthodox Christian worship. Incense is burned within the liturgy in censors which swing from three chains, each strung with bells, meaning that with each pendular swing of the censor a tintinnabulation of sound accompanies the plume of sweetly scented smoke. While local tradition varies on some aspects of this, this kind of censor is usually only swung by a member of the clergy. When the censor is filled, a priest (or bishop, if present) blesses the incense, and then the priest or deacon begins the censing. At the beginning of most services, a deacon will do what is called a 'great censing,' wherein he (all clergy are male) leaves the altar and censes the entire nave – walking up and down each side of the room, censing each person and icon (or each group of people and groups of icons, depending on the crowd). There are also various kinds of 'little censing' that may, for example, include only swinging the censor around the Holy Table or other specific locations within the temple. When censing is done by lay persons – usually at home, not in a liturgical setting – it is usually done with a small hand-held censor, without bells. In the Orthodox communities within which I have conducted research over the years, individuals tend to use incense in the home as part of their personal devotion on feast days or other special occasions. Though some use it to add a little 'extra something' to their prayers, when they are feeling in need of extra solace or awaiting an answer to prayer.

Talking about how incense is performed and interpreted can be difficult, as there is quite some variety across communities, and even within a single parish, as to the specific patterns of understanding and use.[5] However, during a great censing, as the deacon circles around the temple, either walking down the aisles of the church (if the temple has set seating) or weaving his way through the crowds (if the temple is open-floor), the people often turn and face the deacon as he lifts the censor and swings it in their direction. Almost universally, the Orthodox Christian will bow towards the censor – sometimes into the plumes of smoke, if at a short distance. In many communities, the people also cross themselves, as if to receive and seal the blessing of the incense. A little censing usually focuses on the objects and spaces used for preparing the Eucharist. The clergy will circle the Holy Table and cense the table of preparation, upon which the bread and wine await their ritual transformation. While the censor is lit, it is also used to perfume the fabric veils which are set over the utensils holding the bread and wine. Between the two formal patterns of censing, there is a striking parallelism to the ancient medicinal and mortuary custom of incense usage. It is difficult to know if this is an accident of history, or an actual skeuomorph, but it is important to note that the 'great censing' follows the pattern of incense burning for general, preventative medicine, and the 'little censings' are done in the mortuary settings of eucharistic preparation and memorial.

---

5 For a discussion of variation in the aesthetics of practice within the Orthodox Church, see Carroll (2017a).

When speaking to people about the use of incense, clergy and laity alike tend to draw upon a couple sets of images for their explanation. The first is the imagistic language – as seen earlier in the tradition following the Apocalypse of John – likening incense as prayer. The metonymic link follows Psalm 141, which starts 'Let my prayer arise in thy sight as incense, and let the lifting up of my hands be an evening sacrifice.' This is a hymn sung throughout the period of Lent and carries a strong overtone of supplicatory prayer. Drawing on this motif, people interpret the upward movement of the smoke as a visualisation of their prayer – or, at times, a visual reminder to pray.

The second explanation that is often given builds on the fact that the deacon, as he makes his rounds during the great censing, treats people and icons the same. Towards each he swings the censor, sending up a plume of smoke before their face. Within Orthodox Christianity, where iconographic images are everywhere, the understanding of the human as 'the image and likeness of God' takes a very direct implication. Elsewhere, I have argued that Orthodox self-cultivation can be understood within an arts-framework, such that the Orthodox Christian makes herself into an art-like subject (Carroll 2018). Here, in the practice of censing, the Orthodox person is treated much the same as the (other) icons. As one informant told me, 'When the deacon censes us, he is treating us as icons of God.' Later, she went on to clarify,

> It is like a reminder, cuz we're not holy, but we're called to be holy. 'Be ye holy' [she quotes scripture][6] 'even as I AM holy,' and so if we are icons, if we are living as images of Christ, then we are censed as icons. If we are not holy, then incense reminds us to be holy.

One man, who served in the Altar, and was often tasked with preparing and holding the censor for the priest, took the image further. 'I like standing in it,' he said, speaking of the plumes of smoke. 'It's like a fumigant for my soul.'

In Orthodox Christian thought, the principle of being holy is achieved through a process of purification and, ultimately, healing. While judicial language is sometimes used in Orthodox contexts around sin, the predominant metaphors of sin are that of illness. In fact, Patristic sources tend to link the sickness of the body as related to the sickness of the soul, as a result of sin (Larchet 2002:26ff). This is not to say that sick people are sick because they have sinned, but that sickness itself exists only because, since Adam, sin exists in the world. Thus, spiritual illness is framed as being both an antecedent of bodily illness and a detriment to the eternal well-being of the person. Within this context, it is not surprising that the hospice (and later

---

6 Originally given as a command to the Hebrews in Leviticus 11.44, Peter also uses it as an exhortation in 1 Peter 1.16.

hospitals), as an institution of both physical and spiritual care, began in Constantinople and other Eastern Roman cities as places to host and care for travellers and pilgrims (Miller 1984; Besciu 2009; Scarborough 1984). The framework that the Orthodox Church uses to facilitate health, however, is predominantly through idioms of fragrance. This is nowhere more explicit than in the service of Holy Unction – celebrated each year on the Wednesday before Pascha (Easter) – when a fragrant unguent is made for the anointing of the sick.

Discussion

It would be easy to say, 'this is a symbol,' and leave it at that. The ideas of illness and health map onto the feelings of remorse (or guilt, or shame), and the idea of Christ's role as mediator of forgiveness and restitution becomes bundled with symbols of physical healing on one side (as a physician) and spiritual purity and the smell of prayer on the other. However, I think that this short-changes the issues at hand. Yes, human cultures find symbols compelling (cf. Geertz 1966), but why? What is it about incense that is such a compelling medium of both purity and health? And conversely, what does the endurance of incense as a substance of ritual health allow us to know about the human person?

The Patristic sources, as well as contemporary Orthodox faithful, highlight how the person's soul and body are affected by each other, and also each is affected by external things and situations around them (Carroll 2017b, c). The purity of the soul is affected by the conduct of the body, and the well-being of the body is affected by the state of the soul (see Larchet 2002 for a specific discussion about this in relation to mental illness, anxiety, etc.). So too are things external to the body able to help or harm the well-being – and sanctity – of the soul and body. Within my longer work on the role of materials in Orthodox Christian worship (2018), I argue that Orthodox use the material indexicality of things such as textiles in order to help in the cultivation of themselves as art-like subjects. Here, I would like to suggest that there is something about substances like incense and oil that allow them to be engaged and marshalled within ritual healing.

I have highlighted the Orthodox perspective on the person as being permeable and processual (Carroll 2017b, 2018). Karl Smith (2012), in his re-examination of personhood within anthropological literature, highlights a porous quality to the person, such that human formation is done in mutuation with others, not in isolation. Smith borrows the term 'porous selves' from Charles Taylor (2007), but shifts it away from Taylor's definition where porosity (as opposed to buffered) suggests an openness to spirits and meanings inherent in external objects. I would like to use porous in a third manner, drawing on both these ideas. Orthodox Christians are porous selves in Taylor's sense. They acknowledge the presence of spirits (saints, angels, etc.) at hand within the world, in the temple, and with them in life. They also have a sense of mutuation between individual Christians that suggest one person's spiritual state will have a direct impact on those around them.[7] My specific contention here, however, builds on this. The porosity of person, such that things outside and inside have direct impact on each other, and external things are understood to have inherent agency in their own right, rests in no small part on the material porosity of the body itself. Ultimately, the affordance – as Gibson (1979) pointed out in his original coining of the term – rests in the capacity of the substances and the surfaces involved.

In framing the question in terms of the agency (or action) of materials, there are two levels that must be engaged. The first is the biological, or bio-chemical aspect. This area is almost entirely outside my own realm of under-standing, but it is an area of which I think social scientific research needs to be more critically aware. Cursory research into the biochemical sciences highlight that frankincense has observable impact on human cancer cells (Dozmorov et al. 2014) and mammalian emotion (Moussaieff et al. 2008). Aromatherapy and the essential oils market runs rampant with claims as to the properties and medical benefits which various oils 'may' have, and read-ing the descriptions sound quite like Dioscorides in terms of the panacea qualities of these oils. However, it is important to recognise the physical and chemical properties of materials and the potential contribution they have to human sociality. Moussaieff and associates, running highly focused tests on the constituent elements of frankincense and their impact on pathways within mice brains, arrive at a startling and wonderful insight: frankincense seems to make mammals (or at least this specific kind of mice) feel warm and happy. The authors suggest that, with further study, frankincense may be a suitable option in addressing problems with anxiety and depression. This kind of human-material interaction operates within human bodies even when the subject is unaware. Pulled into the lungs or pores of the skin, the chemical elements enter the bloodstream and are able to enact change within the human body. The affordance of the material engages the surface (in this case, the brain tissue) of the subject, producing precognitive responses in the organism. The effect on mood and temperament may be noticed after the fact, but the social agency of the chemical must be acknowledged, and so too must the permeability of the human person.

The second aspect of the indexicality of materials operates in tandem with human cognition. There may not be a hard boundary here, so much as a scale of perceivability and the capacity to (re)cognise the social action of materials once highlighted. Susanne Küchler (2005) shows this in the ways that Cook Islanders employ cheap, non-colour-fast fabric to make their quilts. In a context where the hours of production render the finished quilts highly costly, and the availability of textiles mean they could easily get good

---

7 See, for example, St Seraphim of Sarov's instruction that 'Acquire the Spirit of Peace and a thousand souls around you will be saved.'

quality, colour-fast textiles, their choice to use poor quality fabric is striking. The fact that the cloth is easily ripped, however, such that it can be shredded – straight off the bolt – and then sewn, unstitched, rearranged, resewn, and undone again, means that the ephemerality and variability of the material echoes the social patterns and lines of kinship and adoption practiced within the community. The fact that the textiles bleed and will lose their colour also allows the quilted fabric to resonate materially with the images of flowers in full bloom – the point at which they are most fragrant and almost dead – made from the mosaic scraps of cloth. In this kind of setting, the 'graphic gesture' of art (or ritual) is, as Gell argued, not representational of society, but constitutive of it (1998:191; see also Küchler and Carroll 2019). We must look, then, at the indexicality and graphic gesture of incense.

In terms of the actual process of the material, it is important to note that burning incense is a transformation, rather than an act of destruction. As seen in Dioscorides' instructions concerning soot, burning is an act of remediation (Bolter and Grusin 1999; Meyer 2011), turning the agent from one substance to another. The medicinal qualities still adhere. In the production of the pungent odour of incense, there is also an element of transduction (Keane 2013), particularly in the context where the rising smoke is metonymic for prayer and the perfume is synecdochic for divine presence. Keane's use of transduction assumes a textual basis for the agentive power being moved through media. The writing of sacred scripture, moved via water soluble ink into a drink, for example, carries the potency of the spoken word through liquid into the body. However, the transduction of indexical qualities does not require a textual, communicative aspect. As a transformative act, the ignition of the incense activates the latent potential of the incense and brings it to life. The purified smoke travels heavenward as prayer. It is inhaled into the lungs, and the surface of the body and the surface of the incense become merged, and the qualities (and concomitant affordances) of the incense come fused into the person – body and soul.

The other effect of the transformation achieved through burning is one of making visible the invisible. Andrew Gould (2014), an expert in Byzantine liturgical arts, highlights the fact that incense is an architectural feature of the Byzantine temple. As the liturgical arts of the built environment developed, the importance of how light played within the temple was crucial. Each Orthodox temple is an icon of the universe, and particularly within monumental churches like Hagia Sophia in Constantinople, the placement of small windows circling the underside of the principle dome means that shafts of light shot down from the 'dome of heaven.' In such an environment, incense – as it moves heavenward – catches the light and makes it visible in a startling and new way. Light, itself a recurrent icon of Christ and divine presence, is made more visible via the incense smoke.

The position of the person within this remediation is crucial. The multisensory aspect of Orthodox use of incense builds on the understanding of the body as a site of encounter. As a theological position, the importance of the body has been at the heart of many Patristic writing. Cyril of Jerusalem (313–386), for example, emphasises the body and its place in the divine economy. His teaching, spread throughout his Catechetical Lectures, focuses on the body as a perfectly created apparatus for meeting God through the senses (cf. Ashbrook Harvey 2006:60). The human, with her somatic senses, and the porous nature of her body, such that odours, oils, and food may come into, and be infused and conjoined within, means she is a material being with the properties and affordances easily transformed via such materials like myrrh and frankincense:

> Through smell, it seemed to [Patristic] writers, human and divine could meet – not face to face as distinct realities, but intermingled in a communion of being. Olfactory experience could mirror sacramental reality: to smell God was to know God as a transcendent yet transforming presence, a presence actively known through bodily experience.
>
> (2006:65)

What we see, then, in the materiality of medical substances taken up and used within Orthodox ritual worship, is that the affordances of the *materia medica* map within the social framework of health – both physical and spiritual – and are able to shape and transform these conceptions because of the material properties, joining to and being absorbed within the physical being of the human person.

Acknowledgements

I am deeply indebted to the many Orthodox parishes and individuals that have allowed me to conduct research with them, especially those at St Aethelwald's London. A special thanks goes to Sarah Meitz, who provided very helpful provocations and comments on this chapter. Similarly, I thank the other contributors to this volume whose critical suggestions have been invaluable. Research leading to this chapter has been conducted over several years, under several funding schemes, including the support of the Paleologos Graduate Scholarship of the Greek Orthodox Archdiocese of America and British Academy.

References

Ashbrook Harvey, Susan (2006). *Scenting Salvation: Ancient Christianity and the Olfactory Imagination*. California: University of California Press.

Atchley, Cuthbert (1909). *A History of the Use of Incense in Divine Worship*. London: Longmans, Green.

Athenagoras (1885). A Plea for the Christians. In Arthur Cleveland Coxe (Ed.), *The Ante-Nicene Fathers, Volume 2: Fathers of the Second Century: Hermas, Tatian,*

Athenagoras, Theophilus, and Clement of Alexandria: American Edition. Buffalo: Christian Literature Company, 129–148.

Besciu, M. (2009). The Byzantine physicians. *Transilvania* 6(51):33–38.

Bolter, J., R. Grusin (1999). *Remediation: Understanding New Media*. Cambridge, MA: MIT Press.

Brent, Allen (2010). *Cyprian and Roman Carthage*. Cambridge: Cambridge University Press.

Carroll, Timothy (2017a). The ethics of Orthodoxy as the aesthetics of the local church. *World Art* 7(2):353–371. DOI: 10.1080/21500894.2017.1292310.

Carroll, Timothy (2017b). Im/material objects: Relics, gestured signs, and the substance of the immaterial. In T. Hutchings and J. McKenzie (Eds.), *Materiality and the Study of Religion: The Stuff of the Sacred*. London and New York: Routledge, 119–132.

Carroll, Timothy (2017c). Textiles and the making of sacred space. *Textile History* 48(2). DOI: 10.1080/00404969.2016.1266232.

Carroll, Timothy (2018). *Orthodox Christian Material Culture: Of People and Things in the Making of Heaven*. London and New York: Routledge.

Caseau, Beatrice (2007). Incense and Fragrances: From House to Church. A Study of the Introduction of Incense in the Early Byzantine Christian Churches. In Michael Grünbart, Ewald Kislinger, Anna Muthesius and Dionysios Stathakopoulos (Eds.), *Material Culture and Well-being in Byzantium (400–1453)*. Wein: Österreichische Akademie der Wissenschaften, 75–92.

Chrysostom, John (1979). *Discourse I. In Discourses against Judaizing Christians, The Fathers of the Church, Volume 68*. Washington, DC: Catholic University of America Press, 1–34.

Clement of Alexandria (1885). The Instructor. In Arthur Cleveland Coxe (Ed.), *The Ante-Nicene Fathers, Volume 1: The Apostolic Fathers with Justin Martyr and Irenæus: American Edition*. Buffalo: Christian Literature Company, 209–298.

Coxe, Arthur Cleveland (Ed.) (1885). *The Ante-Nicene Fathers, Volume 1: The Apostolic Fathers with Justin Martyr and Irenæus: American Edition*. Buffalo: Christian Literature Company.

Dioscorides, Pedanius (2000). *De Materia Medica: Book One – Aromatics*. Trans. T.A. Osbaldenston. Johannesburg: IBIDIS Press.

Dozmorov, Mikhail G. et al. (2014). Differential effects of selective frankincense (Ru Xiang) essential oil versus non-selective sandalwood (Tan Xiang) essential oil on cultured bladder cancer cells: A microarray and bioinformatics study. *Chinese Medicine* 9:18. DOI: 10.1186/1749-8546-9-18.

Geertz, Clifford (1966). Religion as a Cultural System. In Michael Banton (Ed.), *Anthropological Approaches to the Study of Religion*. London: Tavistock Publications, 1–46.

Gell, Alfred (1998). *Art and Agency*. Oxford: Clarendon.

Gero, Stephen (1977). The so-called ointment prayer in the Coptic version of the Didache: A re-evaluation. *Harvard Theological Review* 79(1–2):67–84.

Gibson, James (1979). The theory of affordances. In his *The Ecological Approach to Visual Perception*. Boston: Houghton Mifflin, 127–137.

Gould, Andrew (2014). An icon of the Kingdom of God: The integrated expression of all the liturgical arts – Part 12: Incense – Heavenly fragrance and transfigured light. *Orthodox Arts Journal*. 3 December 2014. Accessed www.orthodoxartsjournal.

org/icon-kingdom-god-integrated-expression-liturgical-arts-part-12-incense-heav
enly-fragrance-transfigured-light/

Hahn, Cynthia (1997). Seeing and believing: The construction of sanctity in Early-Medieval saints' shrines. *Speculum* 72(4):10–1106.

Justin, Martyr (1885). The First Apology. In Arthur Cleveland Coxe (Ed.), *The Ante-Nicene Fathers, Volume 1: The Apostolic Fathers with Justin Martyr and Irenæus: American Edition*. Buffalo: Christian Literature Company, 163–187.

Keane, Webb (2013). On spirit writing: Materialities of language and the religious work of transduction. *JRAI* 19(1):1–17.

Küchler, Susanne (2005). Why Are there quilts in Polynesia. In S. Küchler and D. Miller (Eds.), *Clothing as Material Culture*. Oxford: Berg, 175–191.

Küchler, Susanne and Timothy Carroll (2019). Art. In L. Wilkie and J. Chenoweth (Eds.), *A Cultural History of Objects: Modern Period, 1900 to Present*. London: Bloomsbury.

Larchet, Jean-Claude (2002). *The Theology of Illness*. Crestwood, NY: St Vladimir's Seminary Press.

Lascaratos, J., G. Lascaratos and A. Kostakopoulos (2004). Surgical confrontation of urolithiasis in Byzantium. *Urology* 63:806–809.

Meyer, Birgit (2011). Mediation and immediacy: Sensational forms, semiotic ideologies and the question of the medium. *Social Anthropology* 19(1):23–39.

Miller, Timothy (1984). Byzantine Hospitals. *Dumbarton Oaks Papers Vol 38, Symposium on Byzantine Medicine*, 53–63.

Moussaieff, Arieh, et al. (2008). Incensole acetate, an incense component, elicits psychoactivity by activating TRPV3 channels in the brain. *The FASEB Journal* 22(8):3024–3034. DOI: 10.1096/fj.07–101865.

Plutarch (1936). *Isis and Osiris, Vol V*. London and Cambridge MA: Loeb Classical Library.

Scarborough, John (1984). Symposium on Byzantine Medicine: Introduction. *Dumbarton Oaks Papers* 38:ix–xvi.

Smith, Karl (2012). From dividual and individual selves to porous subjects. *The Australian Journal of Anthropology* 23(1):50–64.

Taylor, Charles (2007). *A Secular Age*. Cambridge: Harvard University Press.

Tertullian (1885). The Chaplet. In Arthur Cleveland Coxe (Ed.), *The Ante-Nicene Fathers, Volume 3: Latin Christianity: Its Founder, Tertullian: American Edition*. Buffalo: Christian Literature Company, 93–103.

Tyler, Stephen (1987). *The Unspeakable, Discourse, Dialogue, and Rhetoric in the Post-Modern World*. Madison: University of Wisconsin Press.

13 How photographs 'empower' bodies to act differently

Dalia Iskander

This research is very exciting . . . because [with photographs] everybody is excited, everybody is waking up, no one is sleeping. It is participative. It improves not only the brain but even the soul. I should say soul because . . . it wakes up your emotions inside
 – Participant during photovoice training for facilitators

This chapter documents how photographs are able to excite us, wake us up, elicit our emotions and, ultimately, make us participate in action. In particular, it explores the impact photographs can have on what bodies do in relation to health. The idea that people and material things are intimately related is a rather banal observation in contemporary anthropology. What remains more debated are questions of modalities – *what* shape these relations take, *why* they occur and what *effects* ensue. Pinney (2005) warns that although 'there is a dialectical process of (what heuristically we might call) subjects making objects making subjects' (ibid:269), we must refrain from seeing this relationship as necessarily always representational, linear, and smooth. He argues that the interaction between subjects and objects can also have disruptive and even unpredictable results – in other words, change can occur as a result.

The aim of this chapter is to engage with questions of modalities (ibid:256) and explore how subjects and objects meet and to what effect. Following Pinney (2005), I discuss the potential disruption that can result from this encounter and highlight how photographs are able to facilitate this. By 'disruption,' here, I mean incremental practical changes that photographic objects facilitate among the subjects that make and engage with them. Specifically, in an attempt to bring the material and the medical together for this volume, data presented here show how children from the Pälawan ethnic group in the Philippines make photographs (in a process known as photovoice) that, in turn, make them practice their health (specifically related to malaria) *differently*. In other words, I am concerned with how material photographs change bodily 'medical' practices.

Current theorisation of photovoice is heavily influenced by the work of Brazilian pedagogue and educational theorist Paulo Freire (1970, 1973). Literature suggests that photovoice 'empowers' individuals to make changes to their circumstances because photographs that they take of their lives act as a 'code' (ibid) that display comprehensible but ambiguous meanings about the conditions in which people live that they can reflect on, psychologically interpret, discuss as a group (give voice to), and then use to generate intentionally-informed practical change (Wang and Burris 1997). Following Freire (1973), power amounts to a (psychological) awareness of historical, social, economic, and political factors that affect people's lives and increased control over the decisions that influence them. The acquisition of what Freire (1970) terms 'critical consciousness' (an in-depth ability to 'read' or understand one's world in order to intervene in changing it) is thus synonymous with 'empowerment' in photovoice and is regarded as the nexus for practical change (Wang and Burris 1997).

When applied to photovoice, the implication is that photographs, as objects, are predominantly of symbolic importance in that they make people 'reflect' and 'think' differently about the lives and circumstances that are depicted. This focuses attention on the ways the surface image of a photograph is 'read' for knowledge after it has been produced, prioritises knowledge of the mind, and gives precedence to the power of discursive 'voice' as the means to overcome 'cultures of silence' (the internalisation of negative images of the socially oppressed that have been created and propagated by oppressors) (Freire 1970). However, this emphasis on the symbolic nature of photographs is based, in my view, on a reduced appreciation of photographs as signs (things that point beyond themselves). It glosses over the particularity of these photographic 'codes' which are potentially able to do more than just elicit and transmit symbolic knowledge *after the fact*. Following Peirce's (1931–58) symbol/index/icon triadic sign theory, the relationship between the photograph (the sign vehicle), that which it signifies meaning of (the sign object), and that which understands the significance (the interpretant) is a complex and ambiguous one. I contend that this ambiguity is due to the fact that photographs are simultaneously symbols (whereby the interpreter understands meaning due to a 'learned' process of reading the 'arbitrary' sign vehicle) *as well as* indexes (whereby the sign object has a causal relationship with how the sign vehicle is made) and, unlike most other indexes, *also* icons (whereby the sign vehicle retains common – in this case – mimetic properties with the sign object).

Photographs, then, are not only significant because of symbolic knowledge attributed to what they show by an interpreter (signifier as symbol) but also due to causal properties that transfer between the object and vehicle in the process of their making (signifier as index) and formal resemblances that remain between the object and vehicle (signifier as icon) that allow them to elicit and transmit other kinds of knowledge. As such, photographs do not simply point beyond themselves but *to* themselves. As indexes and icons, they also carry *within* them traces of the bodily knowledge that both directly influenced their making (as indexes) and is retained in the mimetic likeness they hold to that which they show (as icons). This becomes relevant when trying to understand how making photographs, as a particular kind of code (or sign), can potentially affect bodily change.

The emphasis that I place on bodily knowledge that is elicited and transmitted in making and engaging with photographs is significant for health because as Mol (2002) points out, diseases such as malaria do not simply exist 'out there' but are actively *enacted* through bodily practices. In this project, children learnt how to make photographs with their bodies using digital cameras. They then photographed themselves and others participating in bodily actions that relate to malaria. Following this, they used and shared their photographs which communicated these practices in ways that engaged their own and other people's bodies in enacting similar malaria-related practices. As children made and used photographs, they simultaneously engaged their bodies in the process of enacting malaria. Rather than simply encoding symbolic meanings that were open to cognitive interpretation, the photographs that were produced as a result, carried with them and transmitted traces of bodily action and knowledge. As they were then shared and used by children and their wider community members, photographs disturbed and disrupted *practical* circumstances in the present and future by changing the way in disease malaria was enacted by bodies. Photographs are thus able to forge new practical possibilities and identities (Pinney 2005) in the very *process* of their making and use. This is due to their symbolic *as well as* indexical and iconic properties that trace and transmit bodily knowledge between object, vehicle, and interpreter.

Participants in this study did not only emphasise the 'cognitive' (i.e. symbolic and discursive) and practical (i.e. embodied) knowledge that they gained about malaria from photographs as the reason for their effectiveness in facilitating change. Rather, as the quotation from the participant above suggests, other features of the *process* of making, using, and sharing photographs made them particularly effective in encouraging a practical kind of participation and change, namely, the heightened and repeated emphasis on bodily movement – both imitative and innovative – that their making and use promotes; the multi-sensorial and emotional engagement that they elicit from bodies and even souls that make and use them; and the participative or inter-relational and inter-subjective, as opposed to individual, interaction that they encourage between people. By focusing on these features, I offer an additional explanation of the mechanisms through which photovoice potentially facilitates change. I conclude that rather than just promoting the *critically conscious* participation of *individuals*, photovoice also facilitates the *unconscious bodily* participation of *groups*. By reformulating participation and thus, by implication, how to define empowerment, I provide an explanation for *how* making photographs makes children act differently. In doing so, I prioritize an additional nexus for change to that in the current literature – that of *bodily* empowerment.

Critical consciousness as the nexus for change?

'Empowering' people to take practical action regarding their health has been linked to better outcomes for young people in a range of settings (Wallerstein 2006). Much of health-related Participatory Action Research (PAR) aims to empower people by increasing their participation in matters that relate to health. Participation is thus regarded as the route to empowerment and is often defined as the ability of those involved to be made 'aware' of, and have 'voice' over processes and decisions that affect their lives in order to ultimately achieve some kind of 'control' over them (Hayward 2000). As described earlier, following Freire (1970, 1973), PAR is premised on the idea that methodologies that promote participant involvement bring about empowerment by increasing 'critical consciousness.' In time, when combined with reflective action *(praxis)*, subjugated people can theoretically overcome social oppression by taking increased control over decisions that affect their lives. For Freire (1973), knowledge is primarily cognitive (i.e. symbolic and discursive) and there is a direct and linear relationship between how people first interpret and talk about their reality and how they then practically respond and act. PAR has built on Freire's (1973) theories to the extent that critical consciousness has now become 'synonymous with the philosophy of empowerment and participation in public health and community development' (Carlson et al. 2006:838).

Photovoice is an example of a PAR method, developed in the mid-1990s by Wang and colleagues (Wang and Burris 1994; Wang and Burris 1997; Wang, Yi et al. 1998; Wang 1999) that is said to engender transformation through the promotion of critical consciousness (ibid). Photovoice refers to the process in which participants take photos that document aspects of their lives or social realities; select images to reflect on and discuss, raise emergent issues, themes and theories in group discussion; and communicate findings to others including community members and decision-makers (Wang and Burris 1997). As well as being a useful method for a community to gather data and conduct an assessment of their needs, the ultimate aim of photovoice is to facilitate individual, community, and/or systemic change (ibid).

Photovoice has been used in a wide variety of contexts, and many projects report empowerment and change as outcomes (Hergenrather et al. 2009; Catalani and Minkler 2010; Sanon et al. 2014). The vast majority of studies make reference to the seminal works of Wang and colleagues and report increased critical consciousness as a result of participation in the photovoice process and suggest that it is this that leads to what they refer to as empowerment (see review by Catalani and Minkler 2010). However, as Cook (2012) explains, the use of common terminology (participation and empowerment, in this case) and naming creates an 'illusionary consensus' (ibid:2) about what something is, how it is brought about, and what it is expected to achieve. Few studies have interrogated the notion of critical consciousness and provided evidence of how photovoice potentially engenders it and the pathway to change that it supposedly causes. Consequently, there is little in the current literature to support the claim that critical consciousness actually *constitutes* empowerment and that crucially, the kind of participation it implies is the *catalyst* for change.

A focus on the ability of individuals and communities to take conscious control of decisions that affect their lives draws attention to the *outcomes* of participating in photovoice but ignores the most basic way of thinking about participation – as a bodily *process* of taking part (Tisdall and Liebel 2008:2). Taking part in the process of photovoice requires subjects to make and share objects that, in turn, (re)make subjects. The photograph, then, exists not just as a reflective surface image that can be looked at (and cognitively reflected on) afterward but also as a material object that is created and engaged with multi-sensorially. Focusing on outcomes rather than processes fails to adequately explain *why* the making and sharing of photographs leads participants to go from bodily participation to supposedly 'empowered' bodily change. To counter this, I start my analysis with evidence that documents the embodied practice of participating. Beginning with bodily practice in this way sheds light on what shape the relationships between subjects and objects takes during photovoice, why they occur, and what effect they have. In doing so, I point to a potential additional explanation for the way in which participating in photovoice ultimately leads to changes in health-related practices – through *bodily* participation and empowerment.

Looking for participation

The primary aim of the research project described here was to evaluate if photovoice impacted young school-going students' malaria-related health practices as well as those of their families. The study was conducted over 12 months in the municipality of Bataraza on the island of Pälawan in the Philippines between August 2012 and February 2014. Although there has been a 75% reduction in the number of reported cases of malaria in the last decade, the island province of Pälawan is known to be one of the more malarious areas in the Philippines. The municipality of Bataraza in Pälawan has relatively high rates of malaria with cases especially high amongst older children from the indigenous Pälawan ethnic group. As well as documenting what change potentially occurred as a result of photovoice, I was also interested in understanding *how* photovoice engendered such transformation.

A detailed description of methods has been published elsewhere (Iskander 2015). To summarise, I conducted participant observation for 12 months in order to explore the nature of malaria in Bataraza, the role that young people from the Pälawan ethnic group play in ensuring their own and their families' health, and the nature and effect of photovoice in this context.

For the photovoice project itself, 44 participants were selected from four elementary schools in two *barangays* (smallest political unit) in Bataraza (Inogbong and Bonobono) according to specific selection criteria (ibid). I conducted a 15-week photovoice project with these students which was facilitated by teachers from each school as well as two translators, one of whom was a *barangay* health worker. Following a three-week period of training (described in Iskander 2015), participants were asked to take photographs relating to the question, 'what does malaria mean to you?' Each week, images were printed, distributed, and labelled; looked at and individually or collectively sorted; described by individuals through narratives; and discussed and analysed as a group. The final five to six weeks of the project were dedicated to refining what participants wanted to communicate to their family members using their photographs and to designing and making a range of outputs to facilitate this. In this project, young people made a photographic exhibition, pictorial checklists, posters, and a participatory film based on images and held communication events in their schools (ibid).

As a result of making and sharing photographs, a number of apparent changes took place among both the participants who created them and the people with whom they were shared. These have been documented elsewhere (Iskander 2015). Specifically, photographs enabled young people to learn new skills, make friends and be together, feel less shy, feel more able to communicate with others, and change their own and their families' malaria-related health practices (e.g. sleeping under bed nets more frequently, clearing their surroundings from mosquitoes, or identifying treatments for malaria). Overall, photovoice seemed to have an impact on young people's role in promoting health in relation to others (ibid). Photovoice, then, could be said to have had a disruptive effect – it enabled changes to the way participants practically used their bodies (e.g. to take pictures or deal with malaria) and the practical way they interacted with others.

In what follows, I focus on *evidence* of the *process* of participating in photovoice in an attempt to understand how such change occurred. To break this down, I examine the process of taking part in two areas of photovoice. First, the way participants took part in the photovoice sessions themselves – how they learnt to make photographs and how they then used them in sessions, and second, the way they took part in the health practices that they photographed for sessions – in this case, practices related to malaria.

The primary sources of data for analysis are photographs – taken either by me or participants. Mitchell (2011) describes how an important source of data in any photovoice project are the images taken by researchers to document the process – what she calls 'visual fieldnotes' (ibid:136). Building on Mitchell's (2011) work, I use photographs that show what young people were doing and what they looked like in these moments of engagement. While some photographs are those that I took to document sessions, others are images that children took of themselves and each other as they learnt to use cameras – what I call participant's visual field notes. Finally, some images were those taken by children as they documented their malaria-related practices. Together, these photographs help to move away from trying to understand participation 'after the fact' through participant, facilitator or researcher observations, reflections and words *following* the process and instead move towards exploring the actual 'moment of (bodily) engagement' (ibid:153).

Body knowledge: movement, mimesis, and innovation

Wenger (1998) highlights how knowledge is a bodily experience not a cognitive object stating that 'knowing is defined only in the context of specific practices' (ibid:142). As described in this section, photographs showing children making and using pictures and taking pictures of malaria-related practices reveal that at every stage, they engaged their bodies in practical movement in order to take part and acquire bodily skills and knowledge that was retained and transmitted in photographs as they were produced and used. Much of the body movement that children engaged in as they made and used photographs relied on them copying and imitating the movements that I, other children, and even themselves made as described ahead. Benjamin (1993/1999) contends that a 'mimetic faculty' – the human inclination to mimic or imitate – is crucial to human experience, expression, and learning. For him, mimesis is not just the mechanism through which we learn bodily practice but also the way we transmit language, meaning, and culture. However, as well as imitating, children also simultaneously directed their bodies in personal, innovative, and even transformative ways as they engaged in 'new' ways of bodily doing. For example, Figure 13.1 shows photographs that were taken by participants in the first photovoice session where they were introduced to cameras and taught how to use them for the first time.

None of the children in this project had ever used a camera before. In order to demonstrate how to do this, I arranged children in a circle and gave them each a camera. Sat amongst them, with a camera in my own hands, I lifted the device to eye level out in front of me and pressed the on/off button. I then pressed the capture button to take a photograph of what was in front of me and turned the camera around to show them how the image appeared on my display screen. I asked young people to switch on their own camera and then take and view a photograph for themselves. While the images in Figure 13.1 are only a small selection of these resultant images, they illustrate some common themes that have arisen from my analysis of all of these participant visual field notes. These images reveal that young people copied my movements (and each other's) in order to fully engage their own bodies in the process of making pictures. All of the participants are actively lifting their arms to hold their cameras up in front of them and

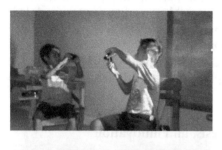
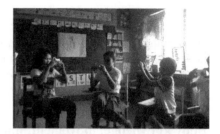
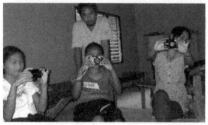
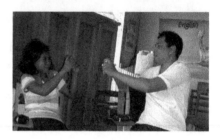

Figure 13.1 Photographs showing participants making photographs for the first time.
Source: Photovoice participants.

focusing their eyes at the screens. Some, however, have innovatively turned their bodies in order to capture something next to them (as opposed to in front as I had done), most notably the two boys in Figure 13.1a. Participating in this bodily way even changed the ways people interacted with each other, and in this way was transformative. For example, these images reveal boys and girls moving to take pictures of each other (Figure 13.1b) and of adults (Figure 13.1d). These interactions are particularly significant as my ethnographic work revealed how Pälawan gender and relative age are important social forces in determining relative status and interactions in Pälawan society. While these factors usually confer separation between groups of people in certain contexts such as the classroom setting, here, the camera brought people together in different kinds of ways. In addition, these pictures show many young people who I had observed (and who teachers reported as) being rather 'disengaged' and 'disinterested' in normal class. Giving them a camera meant that they had to move or modify their bodies in order to actively take part in the process and in imitating each other, engaged in class activity. The process of making photographic objects demanded their (bodily) interest.

As well as taking photographs of each other, almost immediately after learning how to take a photograph, young people outstretched their arms just above eye level and turned the camera round in order to take a photograph of themselves. This happened spontaneously in all groups. The act (and some resultant images) is captured in young people's images shown in Figure 13.2.

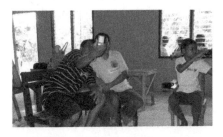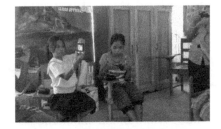

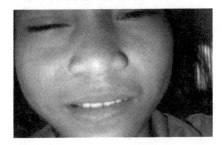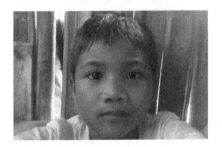

Figure 13.2 Photographs showing participants taking pictures of themselves and the resultant images.

Source: Photovoice participants.

It is important to note that the resulting photographs are not what could be described as self-portraits or 'selfies' in the Euro-American sense of the word. This was the first time young people had used a camera and were consequently not entirely sure what effect they would produce. These images are, on the whole, out of focus, compositionally unconventional (in the tradition of Euro-American photographic styles) and capture rather ambiguous expressions.

The fact that this inclination to make copies of the self happened instinctively in all groups perhaps reflects a broader and almost compulsive human interest in mimicry (Benjamin 1993/1999). This intuitive desire to imitate seems to apply not just to subjects and objects that exist external to us, but also internally, to ourselves as body subjects. There was certainly a large amount of joy and amusement expressed when young people looked at these images of themselves for the first time. Both Sontag (1979) and Barthes (1993) agree that one of the great commands of photographs is their ability to make something stand out – or what Barthes refers to as *punctum* – 'this element which rises from the scene, shoots out it like an arrow, and pierces [us]' (ibid:26). In addition to copying the other, the camera allowed young people to copy the self and produce material evidence of the self being there, practically moving in the action.

As well as engaging young people's bodies in the act of making copies of both the other and the self, photovoice crucially facilitated young people's bodily participation in enacting and imitating health-related practices. Again, this involved processes of both enacting or mimicking already 'known' bodily practice as well as innovating and transforming to enact 'new' practices or existing practices in 'new' ways. For example, many young people photographed each other, people they knew or themselves engaging in 'real-time' malaria-related practices such as sleeping under mosquito nets, disposing of rubbish, taking medicine, and taking baths. In the process of making these photographs, participants enacted practical bodily realities and simultaneously made material 'copies' of these movements (i.e. photographs) that retained a mimetic likeness to these movements. However, participants did not just photograph each other enacting 'real-life' practices. Many young people also specifically staged or imitated certain practices that they could not serendipitously capture. For example, in Figure 13.3a, the image shows young people enacting cleaning their surroundings to deter mosquitoes, while Figure 13.3b shows a male photovoice participant *imitating* this bodily act. Similarly, Figure 13.3c shows a boy who is sick with fever in bed while Figure 13.3d shows a female photovoice participant imitating having these symptoms. Figure 13.3e shows the siblings of the participant asleep under a mosquito net at night whilst Figure 13.3f shows the sister of another participant, pretending to sleep under a mosquito net during the day.

This process of engaging in bodily movements, imitating, and making material 'copies' (mimetic objects) of them was particularly heightened in the process of making a film in which young people used their photographs as creative inspiration and repeatedly set their bodies in motion, 'pretending' to do the very practices they had captured in their photographs. These included disposing of rubbish, creating smoke to repel mosquitoes, and having blood smears and acting out various practices and roles such as the sick role, the role of a healer, and even the role of malaria-infected mosquito (Figure 13.4).

During the photovoice process a whole, young people were no doubt thinking consciously and cognitively about various practices. This allowed them to acquire the skills and knowledge they needed to create photographs as well as to enact intentially-driven changes to their practices based on these photographs to some degree. However, earlier data, as well as those collected from observations and interviews with young people, facilitators, family members and the wider community, also point to something else. They suggest that the practical act of participating was also significant in this process and that the acquisition, enactment, and transmission of bodily know-how was at the centre of how photographs were created and came to affect bodily practice of those that made, used, and viewed photographs. In order to participate in making photographic 'sign vehicles' of practice, children (and the subjects of their photographs) had to enact bodily practice which had a direct causal effect on the form the sign vehicle took (i.e. sign as index). These photographs carried with them and transmitted mimetic traces of these bodily movements (sign as icon) which affected how those that made, used, and viewed them

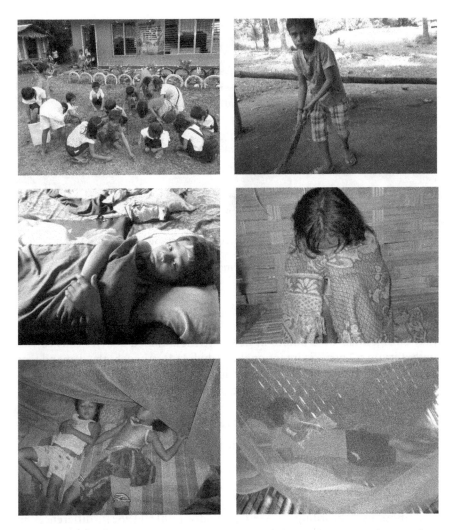

Figure 13.3 Photographs showing participants enacting and imitating cleaning their surroundings, being sick with fever, and sleeping under a bed net.

Source: Photovoice participants.

were able to 'interpret' not just 'symbolic' knowledge (sign as symbol), but also bodily knowledge in the way they engaged with them.

While imitation and mimesis are key here to the acquisition and transmission of bodily knowledge, innovation and transformation are also possible because as Ingold (2000) writes, 'skilled practice cannot be reduced to a formula' and thus 'skills cannot be passed . . . through the transmission of formulae' (ibid:353). Instead, novices are brought to attentive engagement

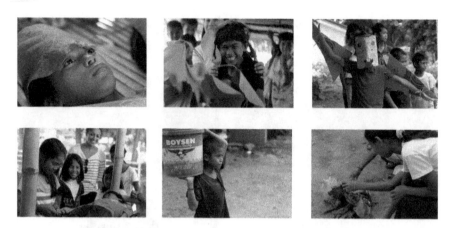

Figure 13.4 Photographs showing participants imitating roles (of the sick, the healer, and the mosquito) as well as enacting acts such clearing rubbish and making smoke to repel mosquitos.

Source: Author.

with new materials that provide them with the scaffolding to work with as they engage their own bodies in new activities. Skilled activity thus carries with it its own 'intrinsic intentionality' (ibid:354). As such, the demand that photographs makes for the body to interact in order to participate in the present has the potential to generate body knowledge which is *both imitative and creative* in the future.

Bodily emotions: taking 'fun' seriously

As well as propelling bodies into mimetic and creative motion, photographs of children taking part in photovoice reveal that making and using photographs also elicited behavioural bodily responses that appear to align with felt emotions. According to Merleau-Ponty (2002 [1962]), differences in behaviour correspond to differences in phenomenologically felt emotion. He writes that it is not just bodily gestures that are contingent on the body's interaction in the world but also 'feelings and passional conduct' (ibid:189). Anthropologists have long acknowledged that 'feelings matter' (Skoggard and Waterson 2015:111) and are an integral part of both human consciousness and behaviour. In this project, many of the photographs from photovoice sessions (see Figure 13.5) capture young people smiling or laughing in the moments that they make, view, and use pictures (both digital images on cameras and printed images on card), as these pictures reveal.

It seems evident that the process of making and using photographic objects elicited emotional responses from participants at both an individual level and a collective one. Ethnographic observation from these sessions

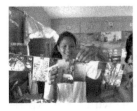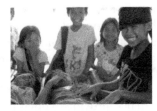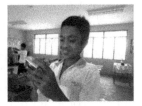

Figure 13.5 Photographs showing participants smiling and laughing whilst using cameras and pictures.

Source: Author and photovoice participants.

certainly also suggested that throughout sessions, young people made a range of 'silent' bodily gestures such as smiling but also made a lot of noisy ones such as laughing, joking, and talking with each other. While I interpreted these indicators as signs that children were having 'fun,' another way to clarify the emotion that these bodily gestures correspond to is to look at the way in which children verbally expressed how they felt during the process. In evaluation interviews, the majority of participants articulated that they felt emotions such as 'fun,' 'happiness,' 'enjoyment,' and 'excitement' as they made and used photographs. For example:

> I enjoyed the first and second weeks when we were taking pictures. It was fun *(masaya)*. . . . I was happy *(masaya)* when I am taking pictures – it's exciting.
>
> Vivian, female participant

Co-facilitators too commented on this feature of photovoice:

> I have observed that the children are having so much fun *(masaya)* when they are doing your project. They are always laughing and joking . . . so I know they enjoy [it].
>
> Denis, male teacher

In fact, one of the most predominant words used by young people to describe photovoice and their participation in it was that it was '*masaya*' or made them feel '*masaya*' – a Tagalog word that interchangeably means 'fun' and 'happy' and thus corresponds to both the object (fun) and the effect on the subject (happy). This emotional *bodily* engagement that images facilitated extended to the way in which photographs were reacted to by peers and family members who, upon seeing photographs of themselves, their children or other community members also smiled, laughed, joked, and enthusiastically expressed their feelings of being *masaya* in both their words and bodily gestures.

A lecture by Hampshire (2012) questioned why a detailed description of fun is left out of much research that purports to be so and stressed the need for researchers to be more focused on and critically reflexive about fun in their work. Fun is certainly mentioned in many studies about photovoice and more generally in participatory research with young people (Fournier, Bridge et al. 2014). Moletsane et al. (2007) go further by directly acknowledging the 'large and significant element of "having fun"' (ibid:21) in photovoice and report that it provided young people with a fun experience that ultimately allowed them to engage in the serious issue of HIV and AIDS, take action, and have an enhanced sense of agency and self-efficacy. Although frequently mentioned, and sometimes strongly emphasised, as in the case of Moletsane et al. (2007), fun is often described as if it were a universal, taken-for-granted phenomenon. It is rarely theorised or analysed as an anthropological concept that is operationalised and looked at cross-culturally.

In terms of *what* fun is in this particular context, when used as a noun, it seems to describe various positive emotions that were elicited in the photovoice process and mentioned above such as excitement, joy, and happiness. Fun appears to be a constellation of feelings and experiences that manifest as bodily gestures such as smiling and laughing as we see in the images in Figure 13.5. The young people here do not just think fun (as in verbally express it or cognitively experience it) but *feel* it – their bodies enact fun. Feelings and emotions are not simply functions of thought but rather are our 'thoughts embodied' (Rosaldo 1984:138). As Macdonald (2007) also points out, in the Pälawan context, happiness and joy and regularly paired with noise and clamour in contrast to the silence and solitude that is often associated with loss, mourning, and unhappiness. In this context, having fun is an obtainable and, more significantly, culturally desirable thing to do. Jesting and joking in particular characterises much of social interaction and are important features of social bonding. From my own fieldwork, I learnt that most meetings between people involve a period of customary joking, and Macdonald (2007) goes as far as to say that the ultimate expression of social life for the Pälawan is laughter (ibid:133).

Here, fun may have made photovoice a 'culturally compelling strategy' (Panter-Brick, Clarke et al. 2006). However, it is important to note that the bodily indicators and manifestations interpreted as signs of fun may have different meanings in different contexts. While a smile here may have largely indicated positive feelings, some images also reveal young people smiling in situations where they also seemed embarrassed or shy. Anthropological insights suggest that the emotions conveyed in a smile are in no way universal (Nanda and Warms 2007) and suggest that more careful examination of bodily or verbal expression is needed in order to situate emotions in locally relevant contexts.

Finally, it is important to consider why it matters that participating in photovoice is fun. Young people reported that photovoice was fun for many reasons as they participated in activities that they enjoyed such as playing games, using new equipment, learning new skills, making and using photographs, drawing, acting, and so forth. These are features that are and can be incorporated into many participatory research strategies apart from photovoice. However, what is significant about photovoice is that it is highly sensorially captivating. As described ahead, making and using photographs requires bodily engagement of all of the senses including that of emotion. Photographs, as objects, offer a rather unique method for achieving and transmitting such multisensory and emotive engagement. Rather than simply being an outcome of the research process or an important way to hold young people's engagement (Moletsane, de Lange et al., 2007), bodily participation that is fun could be significant in explaining the *mechanisms* through which photovoice brings about practical change. More research would be needed to get a clearer sense of what fun is, how it plays out in this (and other) contexts, and what affect it can have on transforming practice.

Body relationships: inter-relationships and the inter-subjective

As already demonstrated to some extent earlier, as a process, photovoice requires the body to engage with a whole host of 'others,' including photographs and other people. These relationships were also captured by the images taken during the photovoice process. For example, once young people learnt how to make photographs, the printed material objects became the main focus of sessions and interactions. Photographic objects themselves (as opposed to the content they display) are important because, as Edwards and Hart (2004) explain,

> Photographs exist materially in our world as chemical deposits on paper, as images mounted on a multitude of different sized, shaped, coloured and decorated cards, as subject to additions on their surface or as drawing their meaning from presentational forms such as frames and albums.
>
> (ibid:1)

As such, bodies engage with the whole object and not just the surface image.

The pictures in Figure 13.6 were taken by me and show young people from two groups looking at their own photographs the first time they have been printed and distributed. Young people's eyes are intently fixed on the objects, and viewers seem fully engaged in the act of looking. Some children are shown smiling, but all certainly look like they are furrowing their brows as they concentrate on the images. However, what is important here is that the interaction young people are having with photographs cannot be reduced to a visual comprehension of the surface image alone. The objects are not just looked at by the eyes but *perceived* by whole multisensory bodies. The

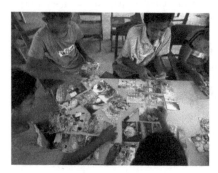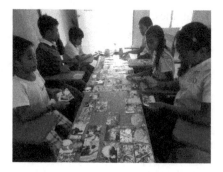

Figure 13.6 Photographs showing participants looking at their own pictures for the first time.

Source: Author.

act of looking cannot really be separated here from the act of touching the paper, as all the young people are handling their images, bending their fingers around them. Rather than being motionless, young people are shown to be in movement as their arms move the objects around on the wooden table and their heads and backs tilt towards them. The photograph has, in this way, grabbed the attention of onlookers' bodies (not just their minds).

The relationship children had with photographs also affected the relationships they had with each other. For example, the first time young people used pictures in an exercise, I asked them to analyse and organise images made by others into similar and create a small exhibition of select images. Initially, I asked participants to appoint a group leader to lead the task. Some young people volunteered themselves for the role, whereas others were appointed by the group. The creation of roles within the group resulted in leaders directly engaging much more with the images themselves compared with other members who took more of a back seat. This is reflected in some of the pictures from this session which are shown in Figure 13.7.

In these images, we can see 'leaders' engaging directly with photographs as they sort through them, hold them up to show to the rest of the group, place them into groups, and stick them onto walls. Many other young people in the group, rather than being attentive to what is going on, appear to be bored, disengaged, or are simply idly standing back passively observing the action. In this case, direct multisensory engagement with material objects was only for a limited few, and participation, therefore, conferred 'power' to the some whilst simultaneously stripping it away from others.

When it came to contextualising the images to the rest of class, it was noticeable that the children who were not leaders struggled to give articulated meaning to images, nor could they explain the rationale behind their inclusion in their exhibition. This suggests that there is a link between the bodily act of engagement, meaning-making, and the potential for images to

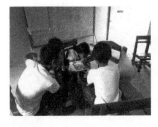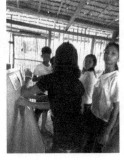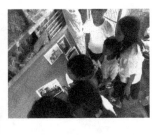

Figure 13.7 Photographs showing participants using pictures in sessions.

Source: Author.

have different kinds of bodily affects. Being present but passive in terms of bodily engagement with images was arguably not enough to allow young people to come to an understanding of what pictures were showing, what they 'meant' and be a beneficiary of all the 'work' that they were doing.

Following on from this session, I no longer asked participants to appoint leaders in group work, and this was much more successful in allowing more young people to actively participate (i.e. engage with images) in sessions. When it came to looking at their own pictures, the fact that the images were printed out meant young people had to actively sort and share pictures and were all required to put up their own exhibition pictures. Furthermore, young people actively engaged in contextualising their images and took part in the act of writing or thinking about them and then communicating narratives about them to the class. These aspects of engagement are shown in the images shown in Figure 13.8.

When engaged in the act of communicating significance of their images to others, young people stood in front of the group and spoke out, often holding pieces of paper with their notes in their hands. Young people found this to be the hardest aspect of photovoice to begin with. However, over time, and with repeated practice, they felt more and more able and comfortable adding words to their images. In fact, young people reported that the skills of 'speaking in front of people' or 'standing at the front' were things they most enjoyed and felt they learnt in the process. The act of meaning-making involved bodily actions like speaking in front of others, listening to others, and explaining images through actions (like pointing). In fact, 'being together' was a sentiment that young people expressed as being a positive feature and outcome of their involvement in the project. This is particularly significant in Pälawan culture where being together is socially desirable and is linked to happiness, success, and harmony.

As material objects, then, the photographs produced in photovoice become important, not simply because of their 'symbolic meaning' (i.e.

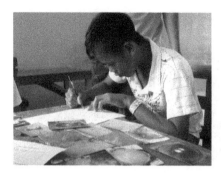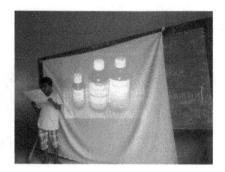

Figure 13.8 Photographs showing participants contextualising their images.
Source: Author.

because of the content they convey through their surface images) but also because of their role as social agents that 'do' (Gell 1998) certain things to bodies. Here, we see how in this project children engaged with photographs in a multisensory way that affected not just their relationships with these objects but also their relationships with each other.

Discussion

Data presented in this chapter highlight the need for researchers to refocus their attention on the specific ways that their methods and strategies facilitate participation as a *process, look for* it in different kinds of data, and define *what* it looks like. I have documented how the process of making and perceiving photographs is an embodied process that participants engage in multi-sensorially at various stages of photovoice. This helps to answer the question of how photovoice encourages a particular kind of bodily participation and specifically how material photographs then change bodily 'medical' practices.

Understanding why people do what they do, and by extension, how this might potentially be altered, is at the core of anthropology. Debate centres on the relationship between society (structure) and people (agency) and, crucially, what is it that mediates the two. Significantly, the mediating role of unconscious is a somewhat controversial topic in the social sciences (Akram 2013) and is often neglected in health-related research. However, I contend that it is an area that deserves more attention. As described earlier, the current literature on photovoice focuses on the supposed symbolic meaning of the content that is contained in the surface image of the photographs. Current thinking is that through taking part in consciously reflecting on meanings that ultimately lie outside of photographic signs, participants are empowered to make consciously led practical changes to their bodily practices. Participation and empowerment are thus primarily conceived of as cognitive functions. I suggest instead that facilitating *unconscious* practice could be an equally compelling explanation for how and why photographs make people act differently. It is important to note, as Akram (2013) does, that this change in emphasis does not exclude agent's capacity for reflexive, intentional, and conscious choices. Rather, it affords the unconscious a more active role in agency and sits alongside (not in conflict with) reflexivity and intentional action (ibid).

Here, I contend that photographs had a potentially transformative effect, not just because they made participants consciously think differently about malaria and their practices in relation to it (i.e. by raising critical consciousness) as is emphasised in the current literature but also because it also made them unconsciously *practice* differently. The emphasis placed on the 'symbolism' of photographs is no doubt due to what Hegel (1977) describes as the process of objectification whereby 'everything that we create has, by virtue of that act, the potential to appear, and to become, alien to us' (cited in Miller 2005:8). With this alienability comes an understandable focus on the apparent arbitrariness between the signifier and the signified which gives way for the possibility of the interpreter being able to 'read' different meanings from the same sign vehicle. However, this focus on the cognitive symbolic interpretation and manipulation of photographs ignores the crucial fact that in photovoice, participants (sign objects) are making their own photographs (sign vehicles) of their lives and therefore interacting in a fully embodied way in order to create these mimetic objects which carry with them indexical and iconic properties of bodily knowledge. As a result of engaging with these signs (sign interpretants), bodily know-how is used and generated (as well as 'voice'). In this chapter, I suggest that it is precisely the inalienability of subjects and the objects that facilitates change here. In other words, photovoice might be effective because, if photographs are objects *made by subjects*, then the process of making and using them is simultaneously an evolving process of making and using the body subject (and *vice versa*). As Pink (2009) points out, scholars seem generally agreed that the 'transmission of knowledge should be seen as a social, participatory and embodied process' (ibid:14). By focusing on the practical and bodily features of participation, I suggest that in making photographic objects, participants gained not just cognitive, but also practical, bodily knowledge that made them 'do' malaria differently. In doing so, I suggest an additional nexus for change – that of *bodily* empowerment.

References

Akram, S. (2013). Fully unconscious and prone to habit: The characteristics of agency in the structure and agency dialectic. *Journal for the Theory of Social Behaviour* 43(1):45–65.

Barthes, R. (1993). *Camera Lucida: Reflections of Photography*. Trans Richard Howard. London: Vintage.

Benjamin, W. (1993/1999). *On the Mimetic Faculty: Walter Benjamin: Selected Writings.* Ed. M. Jennings, W.H. Eiland and G. Smith. Cambridge, MA: Harvard University Press.

Carlson, E. D., J. Engebretson, et al. (2006). Photovoice as a social process of critical consciousness. *Qualitative Health Research* 16(6):836–852.

Catalani, C. and M. Minkler (2010). Photovoice: A review of the literature in health and public health. *Health Education & Behavior* 37(3):424–451.

Cook, T. (2012). Where participatory approaches meet pragmatism in funded (health) research: The challenge of finding meaningful spaces. *Forum: Qualitative Social Research Sozialforschung* 13(1):Art. 18.

Edwards, E. and J. Hart (2004). *Photographs Objects Histories: On the Materiality of Images.* London: Routledge.

Fournier, B., A. Bridge, A. P. Kennedy, A. Alibhai, and J. Konde-Lule (2014). Hear our voices: A Photovoice project with children who are orphaned and living with HIV in a Ugandan group home. *Children and Youth Services Review* 45:55–63.

Freire, P. (1970). *Pedagogy of the Oppressed.* New York: Continuum.

Freire, P. (1973). *Education for Critical Consciousness.* New York: Seabury.

Gell, A. (1998). *Art and Agency: An Anthropological Theory.* Oxford: Clarendon Press.

Hampshire, K. (2012). Lecture on 'Ethics and reflexivity in fieldwork'. F. Interpretation. Durham.

Hayward, C. R. (2000). *De-facing Power.* Cambridge: Cambridge University Press.

Hegel, G. W. F. (1977). *Phenomenology of Spirit.* Oxford: Clarendon Press.

Hergenrather, K. C., S. D. Rhodes, et al. (2009). Photovoice as community-based participatory research: A qualitative review. *American Journal of Health Behavior* 33(6):686–698.

Ingold, T. (2000). *The Perception of the Environment.* London: Routledge.

Iskander, D. (2015). Re-imaging malaria in the Philippines: How photovoice can help to re-imagine malaria. *Malaria Journal* 14(1):257.

Macdonald, D., J-H., (2007). *Uncultural Behavior, an Anthropological Investigation of Suicide in the Southern Philippines.* Honolulu: University of Hawai'i Press.

Merleau-Ponty, M. (2002 [1962]). *The Phenomenology of Perception.* London: Routledge.

Miller, D. (2005). *Materiality.* Durham: Duke University Press.

Mitchell, C. (2011). *Doing Visual Research.* London: Sage.

Mol, A. (2002). *The Body Multiple: Ontology in Medical Practice.* Durham: Duke University Press.

Moletsane, R., N. de Lange, et al. (2007). Photo-voice as a tool for analysis and activism in response to HIV and AIDS stigmatisation in a rural KwaZulu-Natal school. *Journal of Child & Adolescent Mental Health* 19(1):19–28.

Panter-Brick, C., S. Clarke, et al. (2006). Culturally compelling strategies for behaviour change: A social ecology model and case study in malaria prevention. *Social Science & Medicine* 62(11):2810–2825.

Peirce, C. (1931–58). *Collected Papers of Charles Sanders Peirce, Vols. 1–8.* Ed. C. Hartshorne, P. Weiss and A. W. Burks. Cambridge, MA: Harvard University Press.

Pink, S. (2009). *Doing Sensory Ethnography.* London: SAGE.

Pinney, C. (2005). Things Happen: Or, From Which Moment Does That Object Come? In D. Miller (Eds.), *Materiality.* Durham: Duke University Press.

Rosaldo, M. (1984). Toward an Anthropology of Self and Feeling. In R. A. Shweder and R. A. Levine (Eds.), *Culture theory: Essays on Mind, Self, and Emotion*. Cambridge: Cambridge University Press.

Sanon, M.-A., R. A. Evans-Agnew et al. (2014). An Exploration of Social Justice Intent in Photovoice Research Studies: From 2008 to 2013. *Nursing Inquiry* 21(3): 212–226.

Skoggard, I. and A. Waterson, (2015). Introduction: Toward an Anthropology of Affect and Evocative Ethnography. *Anthropology of Consciousness* 2(26):109–120.

Sontag, S. (1979). *On Photography*. New York: Penguin.

Tisdall, E. K. M. and M. Liebel (2008). Theorising Children's Participation in Collective Decision Making. In *Children's Participation in Decision Making: Exploring Theory, Policy and Practice Across Europe for the European Science Foundation Seminar*. Berlin: o. L. a. t. J. a. Accessed www.childhoodstudies.ed.ac.uk/research/Tisdall+Liebel%20Overview%20Paper.pdf.

Wallerstein, N. (2006). *What is the Evidence on Effectiveness of Empowerment to Improve Health?* Copenhagen: W. R. O. f. E. s. H. E. Network.

Wang, C. and M. A. Burris (1994). Empowerment through Photo Novella – Portraits of Participation. *Health Education Quarterly* 21(2):171–186.

Wang, C. and M. A. Burris (1997). Photovoice: Concept, methodology, and use for participatory needs assessment. *Health Education & Behavior* 24(3):369–387.

Wang, C. C. (1999). Photovoice: A participatory action research strategy applied to women's health. *Journal of Women's Health* 8(2):185–192.

Wang, C. C., W. K. Yi, et al. (1998). Photovoice as a participatory health promotion strategy. *Health Promotion International* 13(1):75–86.

Wenger, E. (1998). *Communities of Practice: Learning, Meaning, and Identity*. Cambridge: Cambridge University Press.

Part IV

Responses

Response
Medical materialities, (post)genomics, and the biosocial

Sahra Gibbon

This edited collection fills an important gap in the dialogue between material culture and medical anthropology, enabling critical reflection on sub-disciplinary differences whilst also creating parameters for generating new and productive synergies. It is a timely and important intervention.

This collection foregrounds 'material affordances' in framing a focus on medical materialities that is informed, as the editors outline in this volume's Introduction, by the historical legacies and cross-fertilisation of ideas in social anthropology, STS, material and medical anthropology. It also aims to reconfigure the content and parameters of cross- and interdisciplinary discussions concerning agency, embodiment, identity, and social relations in contexts of health and illness. Questions of scale come into sharp focus here as papers in the collection zoom in on the quotidian: where tea, government forms, soya beans, or water filtration reveal the uneven, lived textures and practices of health or medicine, even as they enfold a wider biopolitics of how care, bodies, and publics are being constituted. At the same time, clinical contexts and medical technologies move in (and importantly) often *out* of focus in this collection. This illuminates the porous borders and multiple terrains of social life through which diverse objects (and their material properties) of health and medicine traverse, from education programmes to religious movements and urban planning.

While the turn to medical materialities is a timely and an important intervention, I wonder too about the ongoing challenges and even potential dangers in these moves to think through, and with, material 'affordances' in the context of medical practice, health, illness, and disease; in particular, how the necessary movement between engaging with (a) the social meaning of materials *and* (b) their materiality can be sustained when the 'potentiality' (Taussig et al. 2013) of, in particular biomedicine and science, is intimately tied to (often promissory) claims about the agency of the body, biology, or health technologies. Does, for instance, the turn towards materialities in social analysis help to sustain the hierarchical knowledge claims and interventions of biomedicine, or the role of biology? It is interesting to reflect on how these potential dangers and challenges have informed my own engagement with the 'materiality' of genomic medicine and research, but also how these are now shape-shifting as genomics segue into the terrain of post-genomics, bringing new opportunities for how anthropology might engage with medical materialities.

The hype and hope filled era of the late 1990s – where the so-called mapping of the human genome was constituted as a solution to numerous intractable healthcare challenges and where the notion of the 'gene for' held a prominent place in various public imaginaries – provided a complex terrain for an anthropologist attempting to elucidate the material practices and social context of genomic medicine. The 'BRCA genes,' associated with an increased risk of breast cancer, then and subsequently, have, more than perhaps any other 'objects' of genetic knowledge and technology, gained a particular 'presence' across diverse terrains of research, medicine, and social life (Gibbon et al. 2014). Nevertheless, they have, like most other genetic instantiations, proved to be somewhat slippery and elusive objects of social as well as medical and scientific research. In my ethnographic research, they were often absent in the daily practice of cancer genetic clinics, where collective efforts to identify their risk constituting presence or absence were often thwarted by various limitations of resources, knowledge, and technology. Here, the materials of medical practice were clinical family trees, where pen, paper and, most often, hand-drawn histories of disease and illness were co-produced through the labour of patients and practitioners in efforts to parse risk and invest in alternative futures (Gibbon 2002). By contrast, in the context of a breast cancer research charity, the materiality of BRCA genes linked scientific research to practices of memorialisation where names on a 'founders wall' could be imbued with the promise of genetic research (Gibbon 2007).

The materialities of the 'BRCA' genes, therefore, were and continue to be distributed and generative across a range of different social arenas and practices, even as their medical and scientific significance has become less stable and more subject to contestation. The way many social sciences attend to 'objects' such as the BRCA genes, the assemblages and infrastructure that sustains them, their 'absent presence,' and distributed materiality has consequences and may also serve (perhaps inadvertently) to propel and stabilise their purported biomedical agency. In the contemporary so-called post-genomic context – where the parameters and function of the genes do not pre-exist but are only made possible by, and constituted through, the ever present and continuous interaction and 'responsiveness to environments' (Láppe and Landecker 2015) – how we attend to and think through the agency and material affordances of the biological and environmental is of vital importance.

In this context, a turn towards examining the materiality of bodies in medical anthropology (Lock and Farquhar 2007) and a growing body of social science work showing how human bodies are shaped by society and culture (Law and Moll 1995; Wilson 2015) is now meeting an evolving terrain of science. Emerging fields of inquiry such as epigenetics are emphasising the role of the social in not just influencing but constituting the biological, aiming to illuminate the pathways through which the 'social gets under the skin' (Bieler and Niewöhner 2018; Frost 2018). This challenge to the assumed hierarchy of a biological/social interface poses new opportunities for how social scientists think with and engage the reconfiguration of the biological, as a material whose properties and affordances are seemingly only ever made possible through the social. While there is caution, important efforts are now emerging in anthropology and beyond to think with and through a biological which is always 'local' and 'situated' (Lock 2017) and bodies which are only ever 'in-action.'

(Bieler and Niewöhner 2018)

As a result, the claim in this collection that medical materiality is 'inherently biosocial' becomes newly relevant as biology comes to address wider ecologies of social practice and experience and as these are de-materialised and re-materialised in novel ways. In a context where it becomes possible to 'assay the ways that experiences of social interaction . . . have a constituting effect on the biological body' (Frost 2018:901) or where biomarkers become correlated to as precursor of and/or consequences of health inequalities or social adversity, attention to these biosocial dynamics and their material instantiations remains vital. The increasing attention to the biosociality of 'data' as a 'thing in the world' (Nafus 2016) is just one example of the kind of new materialities at stake in the evolving terrains of post-genomics and beyond. Importantly, it is one where the productivity of dialogue across and within sub-disciplinary domains of medical anthropology and material culture, particularly digital anthropology, is already proving central to understanding the vitality of computational forms.

The terrain of post-genomics is just one which is 'good to think' with and through medical materialities as they are framed in this edited collection. I have no doubt that it will propel others in different directions in asking new questions that productively 'undiscipline' assumed sub-disciplinary boundaries and terrains towards understanding the mattering of bodies and lives.

References

Bieler, P. and J. Niewöhner (2018). Universal Biology, Local Society? Notes from Anthropology. In Meloni et al. (Eds.), *The Palgrave Handbook of Biology and Society*. London: Palgrave Macmillan.

Frost, S. (2018). Ten Theses on the Subject of Biology and Politics: Conceptual, Methodological, and Biopolitical Considerations. In Meloni et al. (Eds.), *The Palgrave Handbook of Biology and Society*. London, Palgrave Macmillan.

Gibbon, S. (2002). Re-examining Geneticization: Family Trees in clinical breast cancer genetics. *Science as Culture* 11(4):429–457.

Gibbon, S. (2007). Charity, breast cancer activism and the iconic figure of the BRCA carrier. In S. Gibbon and C. Novas (Eds.), *Biosocialities, Identity and the Social Sciences*. London: Routledge.

Gibbon, S., G. Joseph Mozersky, A. zur Nieden, and S. Palfner (Eds.) (2014). *Breast Cancer Gene Research and Medical Practices: Transnational Perspectives in the Time of BRCA*. Genetics and Society Book series. London: Routledge.

Lappé, Martine and Hannah Landecker. (2015). How the genome got a life span. *New Genetics and Society* 34(2):152–176.

Law, J. and A. Moll (1995). Notes on materiality and sociality. *The Sociological Review* 43(2):274–294.

Lock, M. (2017). Recovering the body. *Annual Review of Anthropology* 46:1–14.

Lock, M. and Farquhar (Eds.) (2007). *Beyond the Body Proper: Reading the Anthropology of Material Life*. Durham: Duke University Press.

Nafus, Dawn. (2016). The domestication of data: Why embracing digital data means embracing bigger questions. *Ethnographic Praxis in Industry Conference Proceedings* 1:384–399.

Taussig, K.S, K. Hoeyer and S. Helmreich (2013). Anthropology of potentiality: Exploring the productivity of the undefined and its interplay with notions of humanness in new medical practices. Special Edition *Current Anthropology* 54(7).

Wilson, E. (2015). *Gut Feminism*. Durham. Duke University Press.

Response
Medical materialities, collections, and artefacts

Graeme Were

It has become commonplace in anthropology to compartmentalise medical anthropology and material culture as two separate sub-fields as though no common threads or dialogues exist, offering little opportunity for collaboration or intellectual synergy. And yet, after reading this compelling book and the range of ethnographic studies highlighting the productive meeting of medical anthropology and material culture, readers could not think anything but the opposite. The chapters offer fertile ground for breaking down intellectual barriers and introduce a new framework from which to bridge two distinct sub-fields within anthropology. At the same time, this book injects vital energy into our analytical toolkit, generating new approaches and terminology to think through the materiality of medical sociality and the materials of the biosocial world.

The contributors in this volume have conveyed well the ways in which the biosocial world intersects with material processes, whether this be engaging with conceptions of bodily substances and medical procedures, or through the establishment of medical infrastructures and provisions of care. Crucial to this project, and which Carroll and Parkhurst rightly raise from the outset of this book, is the question, what is the 'thing' in medical materialities that lies at the heart of this anthropological project? Their first response is to look towards historic divisions in the discipline but to use these schisms to highlight points of commonality. Citing Eisenberg's (1977) key debate on making the distinction between disease and illness as an object of medical anthropology, Carroll and Parkhurst compare this to the recent object of material culture debate – that is, the dialectic between materials and materiality which has driven anthropologists such as Ingold and Tilley (and including myself) to contest (Ingold 2007; Tilley 2007; Were 2013).

While Carroll and Parkhurst acknowledge that these respective debates appear to be fairly atomised in that they are particular to the sub-fields of medical anthropology and material culture, respectively, their broader claim is that the study of 'things' lies at the heart of the anthropological discipline and that these 'things' take on many forms and appearances. Thus, to evoke bodies as material substances is to evoke Strathern's seminal essay on self-decoration (Strathern 1979), or to describe healthcare regimes as technological objects is to echo Latour's work on Aramis (Latour 1996). Henceforth, by putting forward their concept of medical materiality, their assertion is based on their observation that the materials of medical anthropology have not yet been taken seriously enough and that medical anthropology has much to offer the objects of material culture as much as debates on materiality do for forms of medical sociality. The driving force for medical materialities is the recognition that while anthropologists have often pointed to the symbolic and healing properties of objects such as shamanic healing rituals for maintaining or restoring bodily well-being (e.g. Lévi-Strauss 1963), or ethnographies of medical institutions captured in classic works such as Goffman (1968) or Foucault (1973), the actual analysis of materials and their constituents have merely played an illustrative role in anthropological analysis of health and illness. As Strathern (1990) has argued, artefacts are often viewed amongst anthropologists as derivative of social relations and not themselves the drivers. In this sense, there is the expectation that the meanings of medical things can be revealed through a study of their context. The problem is that a study of their social context renders the object in question superfluous and 'they become exemplars or reflections of meanings which are produced elsewhere' (Strathern 1990:171). Thus, this book's project is to restore the 'thing' into the anthropological equation and to do this, the book contributors expand horizons by engaging with key thinkers in the anthropology of material culture to examine materials, objects, bodies, and substances.

*

Having myself worked extensively over the years with museum collections of various types, I have always found it something of an enigma that anthropology had, until comparatively recently, largely focused its analytical attention on ethnographic collections. Of those, charms and talismans were well represented which presented opportunities to understand local cosmologies around health and illness. And yet, whilst working on the collections at University College London, I found medical collections in many different departments, from portable electrocardiograph machines in medical science to pathology specimens in the university hospital. These objects were originally used as teaching collections and became formative of canonical models for research and pedagogy across their respective disciplines (Hopwood and De Chadarevian 2004). Their classification and dispersal hindered any productive dialogue between disciplines and collections, thus reinforcing the schism between the material and medical that this book attempts to bridge.

Looking back historically, however, ethnographic collections were often amassed to enable medical scientists to learn about beliefs and practices across the world relating to health and illness. Medical knowledge in the early twentieth century was understood to be located in the study of collected objects such as, for example, the Sir Henry Wellcome collection that was situated as the focus for an analytical gaze. Opened in the summer of 1913 in London's Wigmore Street, the Wellcome Historical Medical Museum marked the culmination of ten years of collecting that coincided with the International Medical Congress that took place in London that year (Larson 2009). The study of objects, collected from diverse cultures such as India, China, and the Pacific, served to illustrate the development of medical knowledge and through their study, could reveal the prevalence of disease over the centuries. Wellcome laid out the credentials for intellectual engagement with collections: the exhibition was to be scholarly in tone and not for a general audience, professional and scientific in nature, and offer a comprehensive overview of the history of medicine (Larson 2009:64).

If Wellcome's scientific ambition demonstrates how 'an infinity of things' (Larson 2009) was understood to be generative of new medical knowledge, then it holds true that the contributors to this book also support this contention about the potential of the material world to foster new knowledge. As Carroll and Parkhurst assert, while there may have been a loss of analytical engagement with objects (much in the way the Wellcome collection was dispersed in the 1950s), anthropology has now rekindled its interest in the object world so that marrying medical sociality with material processes can be understood as a significant step in the discipline's development to build a more holistic understanding of human sociality.

*

In the final part of my response, I use this opportunity to explore more deeply what it means to bring material culture into conversation with medical anthropology, with particular reference to Alfred Gell's theory of agency and my own research. It is important to point out that whilst Gell did not envisage his own work in terms of its extension to medical sociality, his work did examine ways in which the production of objects and images are indexical of agency, whether as carved wooden idols, curative figurines, or protective shields. As Gell (1998:32) states, 'Wherever images have to be touched, rather than merely looked at, there is an imputation that there is inherent agency in the material index.'

Carroll and Parkhurst productively apply Gell's structural framework of 'relations between relations' (Gell 1998:215) to legitimise their project of medical materialities. They extend Gell's thesis – that systems of artefactual relations mirror systems of social relations in a given society – in order to set up their own relational field of enquiry that encompasses not only the domains of the social, material, historical, and political, but also the medical in their attempt to define medical materialities. Their goal is to establish an analytical toolkit that aims to privilege the workings of objects, their indexical relations, and how they make medical sociality possible. This, in effect, was the original purpose of the Wellcome collections – to study objects was to understand their medical sociality and any analytical engagement would reveal the indexicalities that led to prevention or cure in the realm of health.

So how do objects enable medical sociality through their design and application? In *Art and Agency*, Gell (1998) alludes to this in his formal analysis of Marquesan art from Eastern Polynesia in which he presents a historical corpus of motifs taken from Von den Steinen's nineteenth-century analysis of Marquesan material culture. He uses this analysis of the motivic designs to propose the notion of the 'principle of least difference' (1998:218), an operational logic that constrains as much as offers opportunities for objects to remain within a particular style or oeuvre whilst offering some form of innovation, thus rendering them recognisable. Gell argues that the reason why art styles remain true and coherent to particular regions is because of the principle of least difference: a logic which, if transgressed, risks incurring the wrath of gods or invisible forces and thereby rendering oneself vulnerable to misfortune, illness, or even death. Thus, for Gell, thinking about producing objects concurrently implies thinking about their effects in the social world.

To elucidate further, I reflect on my own research amongst the Nalik in northern New Ireland, Papua New Guinea. I do so because framing my ethnographic research within the paradigm of medical materialities opens up new avenues for understanding Nalik life worlds and how certain objects enable certain forms of sociality based on bodily protection.

My object of analysis is a type of shell ornament known as kapkap which Carroll and Parkhurst may have seen on display in the Pitt Rivers Museum alongside the charms that they witnessed. It is recognised by a circular white clam shell disc on top of which is attached an openwork pattern made from smoothed turtle-shell which is made by Naliks and also across the Bismarck Archipelago of Melanesia. These ornaments, worn around the neck of high-ranking men and women, are indexical to bodies as they bring hard/impermeable/male and soft/permeable/female substances – clam shell and turtle-shell into contact with one another – and secured together by tying a length of string through the centre of each.

Kapkap are person-like, as they attract biographical relations and traverse spatial-temporal regions through exchange (Gell 1998) and mirror the way in which Naliks conceive of their bodies as a composition of hard and soft, permeable and impermeable gendered substances. They comprise an outer skin that fuses with the inner life force it contains within the pattern, which is itself dynamic and animated. The use of white luminous clam shell connotes life force, a provider of life. The clam shell's colour and hard, bonelike texture (after it is heated in the sun) is thought to resemble blood and semen, which are said to coagulate, dry, and harden in the woman's womb to form the hard, white bones of a foetus. In contrast, the turtle-shell is perceived as a female substance, a soft, permeable, dynamically changing 'skin' (Küchler 2002). This association is visually suggested by the kapkap's patterned fretwork and its smooth, malleable surface which covers the clam shell and which changes form as new patterns are carved over the life course as the wearer's status changes.

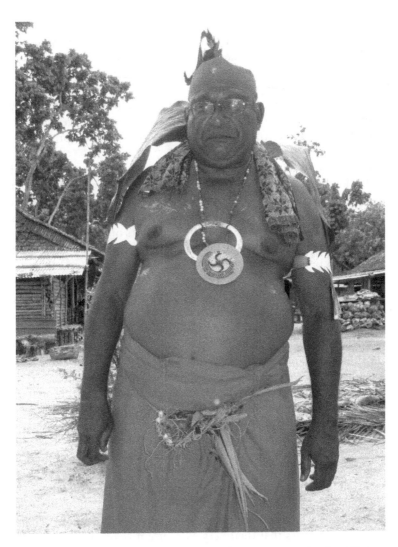

Figure 15.1 Clan leader (maimai) Martin Kombeng wearing a kapkap during mortuary feast, Laraslaba, northern New Ireland, September 2013.

Source: © Graeme Were.

The dynamic skin-like design of the kapkap mirrors the way Naliks maintain bodies and offers valuable protection as a 'second skin' in society where bodies are vulnerable to attack from sorcery. An important property of the kapkap – aside from denoting rank and status – is to protect the wearer from sorcery attacks during times of heightened ritual activities when high-ranking men and women are most vulnerable to attack. Illness and death are never natural: they are perceived by New Irelanders as the work of sorcery, such as malaria, heart disease, and pneumonia. For the kapkap to function effectively, it has to adhere to a clan-based design that bears stylistic and material continuity to ones made in the ancestral past, much in the way Gell (1998) describes for Marquesan material culture. Each design adheres to a kind of template based on concentric circles and symmetry. Difference is expressed through the incorporation of varying numbers of circles, repetitive motifs, and a central quadripartite motif which link the wearer to status and social power, and to cognatic kinship networks which express ancestral relations (Were 2010).

In marked contrast to the emphasis on symmetrical conformity, there were also kapkap made for sorcery which are asymmetric in design. In the past, there was a clan-sanctioned sorcerer who acted as a kind of policeman in Nalik society. The kapkap's asymmetric central design connoted imbalance, and the wearer's role was to kill transgressors of custom, such as those who committed incest or broke customary law (those who caused imbalance in society), by inflicting them with illness or disease (and so restoring equilibrium).

The reason I raise the kapkap as my object study is because it reveals how as Gell (1998) argues, artefacts are generative of forms of sociality. The kapkap functions to reproduce kinship ties and links to the land and ancestral power; from a medical perspective, it also generates preventative health regimes and maintains the body acting as a device to deploy or defend against sorcery as New Irelanders take preventative actions to avoid exposure to sorcery. The type of medical socialities brought about by material culture resonate with many of the ethnographic contributions in this volume which point to the significance of material substances like incense or physical objects like photographs that transform bodies and act as remedies or preventatives to guard against disease and illness. In essence, it underlines why material culture lies at the heart of human projects and how, as Gell (1998) argues, that material processes are in a hierarchical relation to sociality. These material practices create objects that not only can be worn, exchanged, or renewed, but also are generative of regimes of care and well-being in societies that their very existence invokes. Ultimately, a focus on medical materialities pays long overdue respect to the materiality of the biosocial world.

References

Eisenberg L. (1977). Disease and illness: Distinctions between professional and popular ideas of sickness. *Culture, Medicine and Psychiatry* 1(1):9–23.

Foucault, M. (1973). *The Birth of the Clinic: An Archaeology of Medical Perception*. Translated from the French by A.M. Sheridan. London: Routledge.

Gell, A. (1998). *Art and Agency: An Anthropological Theory*. Oxford: Clarendon Press.

Goffman E. (1968). *Asylums: Essays on the Social Situation of Mental Patients and Other Inmates*. Harmondsworth: Penguin.

Hopwood, Nick and Soraya De Chadarevian (2004). Dimensions of Modelling. In S. de Chadarevian and N. Hopwood (Eds.), *Models: The Third Dimension of Science*. Stanford, CA: University of Stanford Press, 1–15.

Ingold, T. (2007). Materials against materiality. *Archaeological Dialogues* 14(1):1–16.

Küchler, S. (2002). *Malanggan: Art, Memory and Sacrifice*. Oxford: Berg.

Larson, F. (2009). *An Infinity of Things: How Sir Henry Wellcome Collected the World*. Oxford: Oxford University Press.

Latour, B. (1996). *Aramis: Or the Love of Technology*. Trans. Catherine Porter. Cambridge, MA: Harvard University Press.

Lévi-Strauss, C. (1963). The Effectiveness of Symbols. In C. Lévi-Strauss (Ed.), *Structural Anthropology*. Oxford: Basic Books, 186–205.

Strathern, M. (1979). The self in self-decoration. *Oceania* 49(4):241–257.

Strathern, M. (1990). Artefacts of history: Events and the interpretation of images. In J. Siikala (Ed.), *Culture and History in the Pacific*. Helsinki: Transactions of the Finish Anthropological Society, 25–44.

Tilley, C. (2007). Materiality in materials. *Archaeological Dialogues* 14(1):16–20.

Were, G. (2010). *Lines that Connect: Rethinking Pattern and Mind in the Pacific*. Honolulu: University of Hawaii Press.

Were, G. (2013). On the materials of mats: Thinking through design in a Melanesian society. *Journal of the Royal Anthropological Institute* 19(3):581–599.

Index

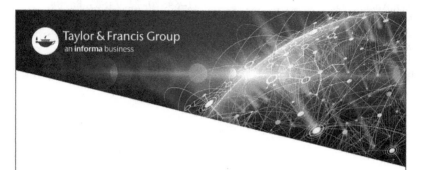